DO YOU KNOW . . .

- How to best deal with a cancer patient's loss of appetite?

- What to do about sexual dysfunction?

- When to contact the doctor about a sleep problem?

- How hope and positive energy can make a lifesaving difference?

- What emotional support you can provide after breast surgery?

- What to expect after prostate surgery?

- How to care for wounds and scars?

- How to help with nightmares or "daymares" about cancer recurrence?

- How to evaluate your own emotional state as a caregiver?

- What to do if you, the caregiver, get depressed or overstressed?

WHEN SOMEONE YOU LOVE HAS CANCER

The Dell Caregiving Guides

The Dell Caregiving Guides

When Someone You Love Has Cancer

Suzanne LeVert

Foreword by Deborah MacDonald, M.S., R.N.

A LYNN SONBERG BOOK

Published by
Dell Publishing
a division of
Bantam Doubleday Dell Publishing Group, Inc.
1540 Broadway
New York, New York 10036

Research about cancer is ongoing and subject to interpretation. Although every effort has been made to include the most up-to-date and accurate information in this book, there can be no guarantee that what we know about this complex subject won't change with time. The reader should bear in mind that this book should not be used for self-diagnosis or self-treatment, and he or she should consult appropriate medical professionals regarding all health issues.

ISBN: 0-440-21664-8

Published by arrangement with Lynn Sonberg Book Services, 260 West 72nd Street, Suite 6-C, New York, New York 10023.

Printed in the United States of America

Published simultaneously in Canada

October 1995

10 9 8 7 6 5

OPM

Contents

Acknowledgments

I have a number of people to thank, for without their help and input I wouldn't have been able to write this book. First, I'd like to offer my sincere gratitude to Dr. Louisa Thoron, formerly of Mt. Sinai Hospital. Her painstaking work on the manuscript provided me with invaluable insight into the science of cancer and cancer research. Should any mistakes remain in this book, they reflect on how much I have yet to learn, not on Dr. Thoron's expertise. My friend Eileen Eaton provided me with moral support and, thanks to her years of experience as a nurse at Massachusetts General Hospital, special insight into the needs of patients who have cancer. Deborah MacDonald's careful reading of the manuscript and helpful comments improved the end result dramatically. I remain in her debt. I'd also like to thank both Lynn Sonberg at Skylight Press and Danielle Clemens at Dell for their steady editorial direction and support.

Foreword

This year and every year, about 1.2 million men, women, and children will hear from their doctors that they have cancer. In some cases the challenges that arise from such a diagnosis are dramatic and difficult, while in others the course of the illness is brief and easily managed. But no matter what, from that moment on the lives of these patients and their families are somehow and forever changed. I know this all too well, having lost my sister to cancer two years ago. As her sister and friend, I helped her and her family cope with the illness every step of the way—through the emotional and physical ups and downs of the treatment as well as through the stages of acceptance and grief as her prognosis became even more clear.

The fact that I was, and remain, a nurse who works directly and indirectly with hundreds of cancer patients and their families every year made my personal experience especially profound. Most of the time, despite my fairly extensive medical knowledge, I felt as overwhelmed by the responsibilities, frustrations, and mysteries of caregiving as someone who had never even heard the word *cancer* before. There was so much that I needed to learn in order to help my sister and her family effectively. And that's why a book like this one is so important.

Indeed, because of my personal and professional experience, I am particularly pleased to see a book written directly to and for caregivers—the husbands, wives, children, parents, siblings, and friends of cancer patients who pitch in and help their loved ones through the course of their illness. Simply having all of the avenues you need to explore outlined in one accessible, easy-to-read book will surely make the job of caregiving an easier one right from the start. Among the many topics discussed are the following:

- obtaining an accurate diagnosis
- finding your way through the medical maze
- understanding what cancer is and what cancer treatment is
- recognizing and treating symptoms and side effects
- helping children and other family members cope with their loved one's illness
- appreciating the spiritual component of health and illness

Even more important, this book makes it clear how difficult and exhausting—as well as rewarding—caregiving can be. And all too often, the caregiver's own physical and emotional needs become overshadowed by those of the person with cancer. While caring for my sister, for instance, I often lost sight of my own priorities, wearing myself down because I didn't feel I had the time (or the right) to exercise or go to a movie with friends or simply relax by myself. Whenever I contemplated doing something for myself, I felt as if I might be abandoning my sister and her needs. What I discovered, however, was that my sister—like most of the other cancer patients I've met and worked with—*wanted* me to take care of myself; when I didn't, she felt guilty and sad, which only increased her emotional burden and sapped her physical strength.

In this book Ms. LeVert provides invaluable tips on how to care for yourself as you care for your loved one, so that both of you can remain as healthy and strong as possible during and after the time when cancer passes through your lives. She'll let you know how important it is for you to take the time—alone and with the person affected with cancer—to "put cancer away" for a while every day: to forget its physical and emotional burdens and have a good laugh, enjoy a sunrise, eat a good meal, just live and live well.

The good news is that the prognosis for more and more people with cancer is excellent. Every day scientists in laboratories around the world are finding new ways to prevent cancer and to better treat the cancers that do occur. Although cancer remains the nation's number two health problem (after cardiovascular disease), we are making significant advances in our fight against this often painful and traumatic disease. I know this much-needed book will make it easier for you to meet those challenges with courage and optimism.

Deborah MacDonald, M.S., R.N.
Nurse—Genetic Specialist
MGH Cancer Center
Massachusetts General Hospital

ONE

Becoming a Caregiver

"I went numb when my wife, Angela, first told me about the tumor her gynecologist found in her ovary," admits Mark Castle, a thirty-five-year-old advertising executive.* *"I think we both did. We went through the whole diagnostic procedure in a kind of haze, and we didn't really feel anything at all until the doctors confirmed that the tumor was malignant. As soon as they told Angela that she had a good chance of beating it because the cancer was caught so early, she went into high gear—learning about the therapies, getting ready for surgery, contacting a support group. It took me a little longer, I guess because I felt so helpless. But I knew how much she needed me, so I consciously pushed aside my fear so that I could help her. It was hard—she went through two surgeries and two brutal bouts with chemotherapy, and my patience and compassion failed us both at times—but she did it, and I*

---

* All names in this and all case histories have been changed in order to protect the privacy of those involved. Certain of the case histories are based on composite portraits of families interviewed and discussions with experts.

know I was able to make life just a little easier during all the hell she went through. Angela's been cancer-free now for two years, and we're looking at the future with real hope and excitement for the first time in a while."

If you're reading this book, chances are someone you love has recently been diagnosed with cancer. Maybe you're the wife of a man diagnosed with prostate cancer, or a daughter of a mother with breast cancer, or best friend to someone who has just learned he has lung cancer. No matter your relationship or the type of cancer involved, you and your loved one have come face-to-face with an enemy—an enemy you've chosen to fight together.

No doubt you've both already discovered how much there is to learn about cancer, its treatment and side effects, and its emotional and physical impact. By now your friend or relative with cancer has been presented with his or her diagnosis, been given options about treatment, and thus has started down the sometimes long, sometimes painful road that, for more and more people every day, leads back to health.

You, too, have begun a journey, one that may be at times painful and fraught with frustration and sadness. But for many people the journey of love and commitment that you have undertaken is also one of self-discovery, personal satisfaction, and joy.

COMING TO TERMS WITH CANCER

Perhaps no other disease of the modern world provokes more concern or anxiety in its victims and their loved ones than cancer. Only a few decades ago the word *cancer* was barely whispered, its ravages hidden from family and friends, and the hope of a cure rarely mentioned. Although every day treatment options multiply and prognoses for many types of cancer improve, the image of cancer as a dread disease persists.

In Chapter 7, you'll learn ways to help your friend or relative with cancer cope with his or her emotions in order to face the future with as much hope and energy as possible. In the meantime, however, it is important that you understand your own feelings about the diagnosis and what becoming a caregiver may mean to your life.

Without doubt you will travel through a confusing maze of emotions as you face the diagnosis of cancer. For a period of time you may find yourself in a state of shock, unable to accept what has occurred. Once the truth breaks through, you'll probably be overwhelmed by a variety of emotions, including anger, fear, guilt, and grief. With patience and understanding you will come to accept the diagnosis and what it means to your future. In the meantime, however, you may feel overwhelmed and confused by your own reaction to your partner's medical crisis.

Because you don't have cancer yourself, you may think that your own emotions are not important or that trying to deal with them is selfish and self-serving. To be able to cope with the many challenges ahead, however,

you must realize that your feelings are every bit as legitimate and important as those of your loved one with
cancer. Only when you come to terms with that fact
will you be able successfully to help meet the many
physical and emotional needs of the person in your life
who is ill.

The course of cancer and cancer treatment itself is
extremely variable and will no doubt feel more like a
roller-coaster ride than the "road to recovery" you've
heard so much about. But there are ways to make your
inner, emotional life work in order to make your practical life more efficient and meaningful.

Making Your Emotions Work for You

In the weeks and months to come you, as caregiver to
a loved one with cancer, will be called upon to perform
a variety of physical tasks as well as to offer emotional
and moral support. This book will help you get started,
and advice from health care professionals and other
caregivers will further aid you. But more than practical
or emotional support from the outside, you'll need to
harness your inner resources to fuel your endeavor to
comfort and care for your loved one. That means you
must not let your natural and entirely understandable
feelings of anger, fear, sorrow, and guilt overwhelm
you, but instead allow them to inform and motivate
you.

To do so you must:

• *Accept your emotions.* You may think that you
have "no right" to be feeling anger or fear since you are

not the one with cancer. Or, if a few weeks have passed since you heard the diagnosis, you may think that your emotions should be stabilized by now, that you should be putting your anger and fear aside once and for all. As tempting as it may be to pretend your own feelings do not exist, this approach will only backfire in the end. Buried emotions will fester until they poison your relationship with the very person you want to help the most, as well as destroy your own sense of self-esteem and enjoyment of life.

• *Reveal your feelings.* Trying to protect your loved one with cancer from the force of your emotions may seem benevolent; you simply don't want to burden him or her with another problem when he or she needs to concentrate "just on getting well." Again, such a strategy is bound to backfire as actions and motives become misunderstood and more is left unsaid than expressed. Open and honest communication between the two of you, as we'll discuss later in this chapter, is the essential ingredient in any caregiver–loved-one relationship.

• *Use your feelings as an energy source.* As distressing and confusing as your emotions may be, they can often be harnessed and made to work for you, not against you. For example:

A period of shock and denial can give you time to get organized and perform tasks that may otherwise seem trivial or tedious when you're emotionally overwhelmed.

Fear often crystallizes important questions you may have about your loved one's disease or treatment, questions you may not have felt able to ask when you were in more control of your emotions.

Anger can be quite energizing, if properly managed. If it does not overwhelm you, anger can stimulate you to push—very politely—busy doctors and other health professionals to answer questions or to focus better on your loved one's needs.

Guilt, when acknowledged, can provide an open doorway through which you and your loved one can resolve both practical and emotional problems. For example, if you can find a way to tell the person you are caring for how guilty you feel when you leave him or her alone for a few hours while you see a movie, you may be surprised at the response you get. For all you know, your loved one with cancer is grateful for the time alone your outing allows him or her, but has also been feeling guilty for wanting to be away from you.

It is likely that you're reading this book at a time when your ideas about cancer and caregiving are relatively new to you. Up to now cancer may well have meant nothing more to you than a headline in the health section of the newspaper or a warning on a package of cigarettes. Now, suddenly, someone in your life has been stricken with the disease and needs your help to get well. Now suddenly both of you are facing enormous challenges that can be met only if you work together.

DEFINING YOUR ROLE AS CAREGIVER

In one fell swoop a diagnosis of cancer has fundamentally changed at least two lives. Indeed both you and the person you love with cancer have been thrust into new roles that you'll be required to play *in addition* to the ones you've already assumed in your day-to-day lives. A person with cancer does not stop being a parent, for instance, nor cease being a lover or coworker or a person with hopes and dreams for the future.

Neither does a person like you, someone who has chosen to be a caregiver, suddenly become a completely different entity. You'll still have responsibilities and functions to fulfill in your job, at home, and in your personal life. You'll have the same victories and disappointments, pleasures and vices, hobbies and duties.

In some ways, then, cancer becomes simply another part of your lives, another challenge to be met along the path of life. Indeed, because of the chronic nature of most cases of cancer today, it is essential that you and the person you care for learn to live with cancer, rather than allow it to define your whole existence.

Without question, however, the fight against cancer often takes so much energy, commitment, and courage that it will no doubt alter—at least temporarily—day-to-day priorities for both you and the person with cancer for whom you're caring. Certain household chores and tasks, for instance, may fall by the wayside while you cope with doctors' appointments and treatment plans. Hobbies may be put aside for a time, or friendships put on hold, while the most acute phases of cancer therapy are undertaken.

Even long-term goals may be seen in a different light as caregiving becomes a priority; buying a new home, for example, may seem far less important than getting the person you love through the next year with as much good health as possible. Understanding that these changes in priorities are temporary—and finding ways to reintroduce former habits as soon as possible—are keys to becoming a successful and healthy caregiver. (Tips on protecting yourself from becoming over-whelmed are given in Chapter 8.)

Perhaps the most fundamental change occurs within the relationship you have with the person with cancer. The new roles the diagnosis has thrust upon you both will alter many aspects—emotional, physical, and prac-tical—of your relationship. Adult children who become caregivers of their parents, for instance, often experi-ence an almost complete role reversal; they were once taken care of by the very people who now depend on them to meet their needs. Similar changes occur within any relationship in which one person becomes ill and the other takes on caregiving responsibilities.

Caregiving as Partnership

The goal for you and your loved one with cancer is to keep these natural changes in your relationship from becoming a power struggle between you. It is often tempting for caregivers to assume responsibility for all aspects of their loved ones' lives, including making the most personal of decisions, in an attempt to leave the person with cancer free to concentrate on getting well. At the same time, people who are ill naturally struggle against losing their independence—to the disease or to their caregivers—and thus may refuse to accept even the most necessary and benevolent of care.

Or the opposite may just as easily occur: People with cancer may become overly dependent on their caregivers, making too many demands or allowing the disease to consume the lives of both of them. Likewise caregivers may expect too much independence and energy from their loved ones, pushing them to live a "normal" life in hopes that this effort will mean that they have a better chance of beating the cancer.

The relationship between a caregiver and the person with cancer is indeed a fragile one. Only if they see each other as equals will it be successful. That means that you must not look upon the person with cancer as a helpless victim or yourself as a savior or martyr. You are both fighters, battling against a common enemy for one positive goal: the restoration of health.

No matter what your previous relationship, you and the person you'll be caring for must both commit yourselves to a new one that makes you full and equal partners. As in any partnership, this one requires three essential ingredients:

• *Open and honest communication.* As discussed above, allowing feelings and concerns to fester will only undermine your partnership.

• *Respect.* Being able to express yourself is only helpful if what you say is heard with respect and understanding. You may not always agree with your partner, or he or she with you, but you must both be willing to accept each other's thoughts and feelings without passing judgment or dismissing them out of hand.

• *Trust.* It is essential that you both remember at all times that you are fighting a common enemy. There will be times when one of you will be feeling strong and ready to fight while the other is overcome by battle fatigue. You've both got to trust that your partner is doing the very best that he or she can to fight the good fight.

Love and affection may come and go. There may be times when neither of you will be able to stand the sight of the other. But if you maintain respect and trust and are able to discuss your feelings openly, you'll be able to mount a powerful fight against cancer together and emerge with your relationship essentially intact.

Becoming a Caregiver

Simply by purchasing this book and taking the time to read it, you've started your journey as a caregiver. As discussed, you're on a bumpy road fraught with many challenges, but the good news is you're not on this journey alone. In fact you have as fellow travelers the friends and families of more than 900,000 people who were diagnosed with cancer this year, as well as the 3 million others who have survived cancer for five years or more. In addition literally millions of other people are caring for the chronically ill who suffer from heart disease, Parkinson's disease, arthritis, and Alzheimer's disease, among many others. And you all share the same goal: to help the people you love live as well as possible as they struggle to regain their health.

This book is written with that goal in mind. In it your duties as the caregiving partner in the fight against cancer are defined and explained. They include

• *Gathering information and presenting options.* Even before the reality of your partner's diagnoses has had a chance to sink in, there are several practical matters you can both start dealing with, including seeking a second opinion, choosing a primary physician and other health professionals, organizing your finances and other legal matters, and garnering support from your partner's family, friends, and coworkers. Chapter 2 provides tips on how to get these tasks accomplished.

• *Becoming a source of objective information.* Cancer and its treatment are complicated subjects, and your partner may often feel overwhelmed by the amount of information he or she must absorb and the number of decisions—some of them life-and-death decisions—that must be made. Although you cannot assume all responsibility for such matters, you will be doing your partner an enormous favor if you learn as much as possible about his or her specific type of cancer. That way you can be an informed sounding board during discussions with your partner and can help him or her sort out treatment options and other issues. Chapters 3 and 4 will provide you with some general knowledge about cancer and cancer treatment.

• *Providing comforting, effective physical care.* Symptoms and side effects of cancer and cancer treatment are widespread and varied. Chapter 5 concentrates on problems and challenges specific to the six most common cancers in the United States today (breast cancer, colon-rectal cancer, gynecological cancers, lung cancers, prostate cancer, and skin cancer). In Chapter 6 you'll find an A-to-Z Guide that describes the many physical reactions your partner may experience as he or she copes with cancer treatment and that also gives you tips on how to make your partner feel more comfortable.

• *Building an environment of hope.* Medical care represents only one leg of your partner's journey toward health. Far less tangible, but every bit as important, are spiritual and emotional resources, from within and without, that may help your partner along the way. Indeed, your partner's state of mind and sense of emotional well-being have a direct effect on his or her chances to make a full recovery. Chapter 7 offers some ways for you to help your loved one with cancer tap into these resources.

• *Maintaining your own health.* As hackneyed as the phrase may sound, you can't do your partner any good if you're sick yourself. It is essential that you maintain a healthy spirit and a healthy body, for the fight you have undertaken may be a long and difficult one. Chapter 8 gives you tips on staying strong and well through the coming months.

• *Accepting the possibility that treatment may fail.* As difficult as it may be to consider, there is a risk with any cancer that treatment will prove to be ineffective and your partner will die from the effects of the disease. In Chapter 9 the emotional and practical issues surrounding death and dying will be discussed.

* * *

In choosing to become your partner's primary caregiver, you've accepted a challenge to fight the good fight against a potentially deadly enemy. It's time now for you and your partner to gather your resources, to become "battle-ready" by getting your medical and financial houses in order. Chapter 2 will help you get started.

TWO

Getting Organized After the Diagnosis

"Overwhelmed *is the word I'd use for the way I felt after my husband told me he had lung cancer," recalls Martha, the fifty-eight-year-old wife of Harry Gould. Harry found out that he had small-cell lung cancer about six months ago. Although his doctors are fairly certain that the cancer has not spread to another part of the body, the Goulds were warned that Harry would have to be carefully monitored over the next several years. His immediate treatment will involve surgery to remove the tumor as well as courses of radiation and chemotherapy.*

"They told us how serious lung cancer was and that it wouldn't be easy to contain or cure it. But we didn't let it get us down. We decided to see another specialist and to fight it as hard as we could."

Martha thought for a moment. "I remember thinking that there was so much to do. We didn't know whom to trust, we didn't know if our health insurance policy covered the treatment. We were absolutely at sea."

With the help of a hospital social worker, Harry and Martha created a list of "things to do" that kept them both quite busy even as Harry underwent surgery. "In a way it was a relief to get organized, to cross things off the list as we accomplished them. It kept us from feeling helpless, and it made life easier to know that we did our best to choose the most qualified doctors and could work with a top-notch medical team. Getting our finances in order was also a great relief; it's not that we won't spend a lot of money to fight this disease, but at least we know what we're doing."

Six months later Harry continues to make progress. In addition to keeping his spirits up, he and his wife of thirty-five years have made some difficult decisions. Together the Goulds have decided that should Harry's condition become terminal, he would choose a hospice approach to his final months of life, living at home under the care of a visiting nurse. Harry has also created a living will, declaring that—should it come to that—he wants no heroic measures performed to keep him alive. "We've made sure we have all the proper papers signed and sealed and have Harry's physician's support. Now we feel prepared for anything and can turn all our attention over to fighting and beating the disease."

"Organization is the key" may be a cliché but, like most clichés, it has a great deal of merit, especially when it comes to meeting the challenges of cancer with energy and efficiency. Just as Martha discovered, the more lists you can create and items you can check off as you go along, the more in control both you and your partner will feel—even when coping with this highly variable disease.

Although each person with cancer has different priorities, there are certain fundamental tasks that should be performed at or near the time of diagnosis. The order in which they are undertaken will depend on a variety of issues, but it is important that you and your partner take a look at the following list. Although the suggestions for actions to be taken are directed toward you, the caregiver, you and your partner may decide to divide up the tasks or perform them together.

The five fundamental tasks include

1. Confirming the diagnosis and investigating treatment recommendations
2. Learning all you can about your partner's cancer
3. Getting to know the health care team
4. Exploring financial options and legal matters
5. Telling family and friends

ESTABLISHING DIAGNOSIS AND TREATMENT RECOMMENDATIONS

Since you're reading this book, chances are that you and/or your partner have had at least one initial meeting with a physician who diagnosed your partner with cancer. If you're like most people, however, after you heard the word *cancer*, you were unable to comprehend the diagnosis fully and what it may mean to your partner's life. And the finer points of treatment and possible side effects may well have been left to discuss at another appointment altogether. Perhaps your partner was told the news when he or she was alone, and then conveyed the diagnosis to you secondhand, in which case you probably have thousands of questions of your own to ask the physician.

It is important that you, as the primary caregiver, understand exactly what type of cancer your partner has and what treatment options are available. As soon as possible, then, and with your partner's support, set up an appointment for both of you to see the diagnosing doctor.

At this appointment try to limit your questions, as much as possible, to those listed below. One reason for this is that a physician's time is limited and, like it or not, you probably have only about thirty minutes to talk with him or her at this time. Second, you yourself have limitations on how much medical information you can absorb during one session. Know that there will be plenty of other opportunities in the near future to ask further questions.

The fundamental information you should receive during this first appointment includes answers to the following questions:

- *What kind of cancer does my partner have?*
- *How advanced is it?* With this question you are asking the doctor how far the cancer has advanced and if it has spread to another part of the body, or metastasized.
- *How was the diagnosis and degree of spread determined?* You and your partner should talk with the doctor about how the diagnosis of cancer was reached. Make sure you both understand what tests were performed and what they showed. Find out if the doctor is

planning to order more tests to confirm the results of earlier ones. Biopsy (the surgical removal of a piece of tissue and its examination in a pathology lab), blood tests, and X rays and other imaging examinations (such as MRI and CT scans) are the standard diagnostic tools to determine the extent of disease.

• *What course of treatment does the doctor prescribe?* Following the discussion of your partner's diagnosis, ask the doctor what treatment he or she recommends. It is important that you ask him or her to delineate the pros and cons of the treatment, as well as outline other options. In addition make sure he or she explains why the specific treatment being proposed has been chosen. (For more information on what factors to consider when deciding upon which treatment plan is best for your partner, see Chapter 4.)

• *Where can my partner receive a second opinion?* A second opinion is not a luxury for people with cancer, it is a necessity. Even if your partner trusts his or her physician implicitly, you should both talk to another doctor with expertise in treating your partner's type of cancer. New developments in cancer research and treatment are happening so fast that it's practically impossible for every doctor to be aware of the most up-to-date ways of dealing with the disease.

Seeking a Second Opinion

All treatment options for cancer are serious ones, involving as they do surgery, dosages of radiation, and/or infusions of highly toxic drugs (chemotherapy). Therefore it is in your partner's best interest to be as certain as possible that the diagnosis reached and the treatment plan proposed by the diagnosing physician poses the best chance of success with as few unwanted side effects as possible.

As well as confirming the diagnosis and further exploring a treatment plan, a second opinion will also give you and your partner an opportunity to meet a new physician who may have a very different way of relating to patients or practicing medicine than the diagnosing physician, giving you the chance to see if another style of interaction may be better for you.

As your partner's caregiver, one of your primary duties is to help your partner sort out the options before him or her, in this case deciding which new physician should be consulted on the initial diagnosis and treatment recommendations. Here are some steps you can take:

• *Reassure your partner that getting a second opinion is not a waste of time.* In all but the rarest of cases physicians agree that it is well worth a reasonable delay in starting treatment to make sure that a patient's case has been properly evaluated. Some exceptions to this rule may include simple cases of basal-cell carcinoma (the most common type of skin cancer), which are easily treated by most dermatologists, or cases in which the patient's life is in immediate danger from a tumor pressing against or invading a vital organ.

Stress to your partner that the first physician will not be offended or surprised at the request but should welcome the chance to discuss options with a consulting specialist.

• *Help your partner choose a consulting physician.*
Depending on the circumstances, you and your partner
may already know whom you would like to see for a
second opinion; perhaps your family doctor has suggested someone, or you've met a patient satisfied with
the care provided by his or her doctor.

For further suggestions, or to confirm that your
choice is an appropriate one, contact one or more of the
following service organizations: the American Cancer
Information Service, the American Cancer Society, the
National Cancer Institute, and/or the American College
of Surgeons (see "Appendix 1: Resources" for addresses
and phone numbers). These institutions provide free information about cancer treatment and keep up-to-date
lists of qualified physicians and treatment centers specializing in treating your partner's particular cancer.

In choosing a consulting physician, you may want to
consider someone who is affiliated with a different hospital than the first physician. In that way you and your
partner will get a chance to see how another treatment
center operates, further helping you both to decide under whose care your partner would be more comfortable and better served.

• *Sort out the two opinions.* It is not unusual for the
opinion of the consulting physician to differ from that
of the diagnosing physician, either marginally or
wholly. In most cases this difference of opinion does
not reflect incompetence on either doctor's part, but
rather honest disagreement between two professionals.
In some cases both oncologists look at the same results
from tests but disagree on what the test results mean. In
other cases tests are repeated only to have the results

differ in some ways from the original tests, therefore bringing the consulting doctor to a different conclusion as to how to proceed.

If you and your partner receive two different opinions about any aspect of treatment, the first step you should take is to get the two physicians to discuss the case together, preferably with you and your partner present. Such a meeting can take place in person or by telephone conferencing. Many times such a dialogue will bring everyone to a greater understanding of your partner's condition, and finally to an agreement on what the next step should be.

If you and your partner—and/or the physicians themselves—remain unsatisfied, feel free to get a third opinion. In this case it may be best to go to someone considered to be an expert in diagnosing and treating your partner's cancer, even if it means traveling out of state. You can obtain names of nationally recognized experts by contacting the National Cancer Institute. Another option is to visit a cancer center run by the National Cancer Institute or a large medical facility that specializes in cancer treatment, such as the Lahey Clinic or the Mayo Clinic.

Once you are relatively confident in the oncologist and the treatment plan, your real education process can begin.

• *Learn all you can about your partner's cancer.* As an essential member of your partner's health care team, you need to become as informed as possible about all aspects of the disease, treatment plan, and especially any potential symptoms and side effects your partner is likely to experience.

This may seem a daunting task, but fortunately, there are many sources of information from which you can tap:

1. Take advantage of the experts closest to you: your partner's physicians. They probably have brochures and handouts that explain the fundamentals of the cancer with which your partner suffers as well as the basics of the proposed treatment plan.

2. Once you've assimilated those materials, head for the library and bookstore. Both will have plenty of books (like this one) that are easy to read, up-to-date, and written for people like you who may not have a background in medicine.

3. Contact the American Cancer Society and National Cancer Institute; both have lots of material, some of it dealing with your partner's specific type of cancer, that they will gladly send you, usually free of charge (see "Appendix 1: Resources").

4. Finally, the sources of information that will probably mean the most to you are people just like you and your partner: other cancer patients and their caregivers. They truly have the inside information on what you really need to know: how to care for your partner, how to cope with fears and frustrations, and where to go to get expert answers. Now is the time you and your partner should locate the cancer support group closest to your neighborhood (see "Appendix 1: Resources").

GETTING TO KNOW THE HEALTH CARE TEAM

Once a decision on the course of your partner's treatment has been made, you both face another choice: Who will become the primary physician treating your partner? This is indeed an important decision, because this physician will become a significant person in your partner's life for some time to come.

Credentials

Evaluate physicians' credentials. In all likelihood both the physician who diagnosed your partner's cancer and the consulting physician are fully qualified to treat patients with cancer. However, it is always a good idea to double-check the physician's credentials to make sure he or she is the best person to care for your partner.

1. Determine whether the physician is certified in oncology by the American Board of Medical Specialties and is a member of the American Society of Clinical Oncology. When a physician is "board certified," it means that he or she has passed rigorous peer-administered written and oral examinations in a field and has satisfied its residency-training requirements.

However, it should be noted that there are many physicians competent in the treatment of cancer who are *not* board-certified in oncology. One reason is that the boards in oncology are relatively new and thus were not available to doctors older than forty-five years of age or so who are still in practice. In addition some doctors in large teaching hospitals or cancer treatment centers combine research with patient care and choose not to take the boards. Other physicians may be "board eligible" rather than board-certified, meaning that they have completed a formal training program in the specialty but have either chosen not to take the exams or have not completed the exams. These doctors are also well-trained specialists able to treat cancer effectively.

2. If your partner's oncologist is not board-certified, make sure he or she comes with a strong personal recommendation from other oncologists, health professionals, or a cancer-related institution such as the American Cancer Society or the National Cancer Institute.

3. Find out what type of practice the physician runs. Does he or she specialize in treating the type of cancer your partner has? Does he or she keep up-to-date on current therapies and medical advances? Don't be afraid to ask questions of the physician about his or her experience. Request names of current and former patients with the same type of cancer and talk with one or two of them about their experiences.

Rapport

Make sure there is sufficient patient-doctor rapport. Competence is, of course, of primary concern when choosing a physician to treat cancer. Once it has been established that the doctor is well trained, however, your partner's reaction to the doctor as a person should be the decisive factor in the choice of a primary physician.

In evaluating the physician's personal style, take into consideration the following aspects:

Does he or she
> Seem warm and concerned about your partner as a person?
> Take the time to answer your partner's questions?
> Communicate in plain, easy-to-understand language?
> Welcome family involvement in the course of treatment?

If your partner answers no to any of the above questions after meeting with a physician, he or she should strongly consider finding someone with whom he or she feels more able to communicate. This isn't to say that you, your partner, and the physician will become bosom buddies; the doctor must keep a certain professional distance in order to provide the best, most objective care. What it does mean, however, is that your partner—and you, to a lesser extent—must feel comfortable with the doctor, since the relationship you all form may last for several years, perhaps a lifetime.

Once you and your partner decide upon the best person to head the treatment team, you will begin to meet the many other health care professionals who will work with you and your partner during the course of the illness. Depending on the treatment plan devised for the particular cancer involved, your partner may be seen by surgeons, oncology nurses, experts in chemotherapy and radiation, and various others who specialize in other aspects of patient care.

Surgeons are very often the first medical consultant contacted once the diagnosis of cancer has been made since surgery remains a leading form of cancer treatment. Although no board certification exists yet for the specialty of oncologic surgery, there are a number of doctors who specialize in performing surgery to remove cancerous tumors. In addition to making sure that your partner's surgeon is certified in general surgery by the American Board of Surgery and/or the American College of Surgeons, find out if he or she has extensive experience in performing the surgery your partner requires.

Medical oncologists are internists with special training treating patients with chemotherapeutic drugs, hormones, and other biological agents. Medical oncologists often assume overall responsibility for the treatment; in other words, your partner's primary physician may well specialize in medical oncology.

Radiation oncologists are trained to use high-energy X rays to cause tumors to shrink. Other names for the same specialist include radiotherapist and therapeutic radiologist. The radiotherapist will evaluate your partner's particular cancer and decide how much radiation is necessary to reduce or eliminate the tumor. He or she will also monitor the progress of radiation therapy on a regular basis. Your partner's radiotherapist should be certified in radiation oncology by the American Board of Radiologists.

Oncology nurses have specialized training and interest in caring for patients with cancer. In addition to receiving basic medical training through two- or four-year nursing programs, all nurses are required to pass a state licensing examination before they can practice. Oncology nurses are those health care professionals who receive further training at a hospital, medical center, or research facility in the care of cancer fighters. Many oncology nurses are members of the Oncology Nursing Society. By and large, these professionals will be you and your partner's most valuable ally within the health care system.

You and your partner are likely to meet several nurses during the coming months. Oncology nurses will assist the primary physician and other members of the cancer treatment team. They are trained to administer chemotherapy and manage its side effects; assist in applying radiotherapy and manage its side effects; and keep up with new technologies (such as bone marrow transplantation and biological therapies) as they evolve. Moreover nurses are usually more accessible to patients and families than are doctors and therefore provide the most consistent emotional and physical care during cancer therapy.

Nutritionists are trained to evaluate dietary deficiencies and prepare individualized eating plans for cancer patients having difficulty consuming adequate nutrition.

Physical therapists are trained to assist individuals who have been bedridden or inactive for extended periods of time in regaining strength and mobility. They can also design a long-term exercise program.

Occupational therapists help retrain patients whose cancer or treatment side effects prevent them from performing the tasks of daily living as they have in the past. Women who have had mastectomies for the treatment of breast cancer, for instance, may need to learn new ways of dressing and bathing themselves while the muscle tissue around the breast heals.

Enterostomal therapists are registered nurses who have specialized training in the care of people who have had surgical procedures known as ostomies. Ostomies involve the creation of a new passageway through the abdominal wall as an exit for feces or urine. This new passageway, called a stoma, is necessary because part of the digestive or urinary tract is removed in order to excise cancerous tissue or to treat other noncancer-related conditions. If your partner requires an ostomy to treat his or her cancer, an enterostomal therapist will assist you both in learning to cope with the physical—and emotional—aspect of this procedure. (More about ostomies in Chapter 5.)

Psychiatrists and psychologists are health care professionals trained to help people cope with emotional and psychological problems. Psychiatrists are medical doctors who have received additional training in the specialty of psychology. They are able to perform medical tests and prescribe medication. Psychologists are also trained to provide psychological counseling, but are not medical doctors and are thus unable to prescribe medication.

As you and your partner have no doubt already discovered, cancer represents a major life crisis that may well require the aid of a mental health professional at some point during the treatment and/or posttreatment period. Do not hesitate to ask your partner's primary physician for advice in finding a counselor experienced in helping cancer fighters and/or family members.

Medical social workers are trained to provide psychological counseling as well as practical assistance to those struggling to cope with an illness such as cancer. Social workers can help you and your partner sort out the many emotional, physical, and financial challenges you now face and set both short- and long-term goals. Many people with cancer first meet a social worker during a hospital stay, but social workers are also available to former hospital patients on an outpatient basis, and to the general public through social service agencies and private practices.

Primary caregivers are people just like you who devote themselves to helping someone they love fight cancer. Primary caregivers begin their training the day they are told about their partner's cancer and continue learning throughout the treatment and posttreatment periods. As your loved one's primary caregiver, you should consider yourself a partner not only of the person with cancer but of all of the health professionals just mentioned and described. By working alongside and in consultation with them, you will help ensure that your partner receives the best care possible around the clock.

Hospitalization

Almost every person with cancer will spend some time in the hospital, either to receive medication or for surgery to remove cancerous tissue. Hospitalization is often a stressful and upsetting experience for both patients and their families and friends, but there are ways to make it easier on everyone, as you'll find out below.

Anyone facing a period of hospitalization should be

aware of the following "Patient's Bill of Rights," paraphrased from the formal American Hospital Association document.

All hospital patients have the right to

1. Personal dignity, privacy, and courtesy
2. Know the identity of all physicians and other health care providers who participate directly in their care
3. Receive full information about options for treatment
4. Confidentiality of their disclosures and medical records
5. Review their medical records

It is every bit as important for you and your partner to form positive relationships with the *hospital* health care team as it is to get to know the primary physician; a friendly nurse who knows you both well can make the hospital experience infinitely less stressful. In addition most hospitals have an ombudsman or patient-services representative to mediate difficulties for patients and families, and patients or their caregivers should not be shy about voicing concerns or problems—about medication, meals, and exercise, for instance—to such a person.

ORGANIZING FINANCES AND OTHER LEGAL MATTERS

Although the last thing you and your partner may want to think about now is money, it is essential that you concentrate as soon as possible on how you will pay for medical care and other expenses during what may be a long and debilitating illness. In addition even if your partner's prognosis for a full recovery is excellent, he or she may want to begin the process of long-term planning, including updating wills and other legal documents and making important decisions about the end of his or her life. By all means, you and your partner should feel free to contact a medical social worker for advice and support.

Financial Options

Financial planning for a catastrophic illness such as cancer goes far beyond the scope of this book, even in the most stable of times. Today, however, vast changes are being proposed by the federal government that are likely fundamentally to alter the way medical care is administered and paid for in the United States in the near future.

Nevertheless it is important that you and your partner sort out your financial options to the best of your ability as soon as possible. Fortunately you have many professionals to whom you can turn if you have questions about your financial situation as it relates to medical care. The first person you should speak to is your partner's primary physician and nurse. They are usually quite familiar with the ins and outs of paying for medical care. Another option is to contact a hospital social worker or a social worker connected to a state or local social service agency. In addition the American Cancer

Society may also be able to direct you to financial planners who specialize in this area.

In the meantime here is a brief outline of some of the options you have available to you:

Health Insurance

If your partner is covered by an individual or group health insurance plan, your first step in organizing your finances is to find out exactly what the plan will pay for. Some plans cover only standard types of treatment and will not pay costs associated with investigational therapies—even if these therapies are suggested by your partner's primary physician. Plans also vary widely on the amount a patient must pay before his or her coverage starts, an amount known as the deductible. Some plans pay for only thirty days in the hospital; others cover many more. Most plans have upper limits on what they will pay toward treatment for a given health problem on an annual or lifetime basis. Some plans will cover certain home-care services, others will not.

Read the policy over carefully and make a list of all of your questions. Before you call the insurance company with any questions, you may want to speak with both the physician and a hospital financial representative and ask them to intervene. Medical personnel are often better equipped than you are to deal with insurance staff and to ask the right questions about coverage.

If your partner with cancer is one of the more than 36 million people in the United States who lack health insurance, it may be difficult if not impossible for him or her to buy coverage now. A preexisting condition such as cancer is often an insurmountable barrier to obtaining health insurance. Other options for financial aid include those discussed below.

Unemployment/Disability

If your partner is currently employed, make sure he or she checks to see if disability benefits are available should your partner's fight with cancer prevent him or her from being able to work. To receive disability benefits, the worker and his or her physician must fill out a form provided by the employer, who then submits the claim to the State Department of Labor. If the claim is approved, some percentage of the worker's weekly wages are paid until the disability ends or a fixed period of time has passed. Please note, however, that state disability laws do not guarantee that the worker's job will remain open until the worker is able to return. For information about the law in your state, contact that state's Department of Labor or Unemployment Division.

Medicaid

If your partner lacks both insurance and the money to pay for care, he or she may be eligible to receive financial aid from the government. Individual states, operating under federal guidelines, run the Medicaid program for people with limited resources. Your partner must call the state or local department of social services to find out about his or her own eligibility.

In some states your partner is automatically eligible for Medicaid if he or she is eligible for Supplemental Security Income (SSI). The SSI program is designed to provide funds to people with income below the federal

minimum level or to those who are disabled. But even if
your partner is not eligible for SSI, he or she may still
qualify to receive Medicaid under the "medically
needy" category. In some states, for instance, Medicaid
helps with hospital bills and bills for inpatient physician
services when the costs exceed 25 percent of annual net
income. Check with your local Medicaid or Social Security offices.

Medicare

The federal government administers the Medicare
program to provide health care benefits for people over
sixty-five years of age and disabled people. This program covers many significant health care costs, but certainly not all of them, and many older people find it
necessary to supplement Medicare with other forms of
health insurance.

No matter how medical expenses are handled, keeping track of medical bills and insurance payments can
be confusing. Here are a few tips to help you and your
partner make sure that expenses are met with a minimum of trouble:

1. Be sure to photocopy *everything* you send to the
doctor, health insurance company, laboratories, social
service agencies (such as the State Department of Labor), or other individuals or institutions involved in
your partner's treatment. Copy query letters, claim
forms, bills, and receipts. Date every letter you write,
bill you receive, and claim form you fill out. Store these
documents in labeled files.

2. Submit a bill for all medical expenses, even those you don't think the health insurance company or Medicaid/Medicare will pay. The worst thing that can happen is that those expenses will not be reimbursed, but you may be pleasantly surprised when something you thought would not be covered is paid.

3. Appeal any decision you feel is unfair, making sure you can back up your claim with documentation.

4. If you have trouble collecting on your claim to an insurance company, contact the state or federal agency that regulates your insurance provider. If you have trouble with government assistance, ask a hospital social worker, or even your partner's physician, to intervene. You may also want to contact cancer support organizations such as the American Cancer Society. Many of them offer ombudsman programs to help cancer patients and their families deal with the insurance companies.

Planning for the Future

As stated at the beginning of this chapter, even if your partner's prognosis is good, the diagnosis of cancer may provoke questions and concerns about the future and how to plan for it. Indeed, as unpleasant as the thought may be, we will all die someday. Before we die, many of us will also become incapacitated by illness and unable to make our own financial or medical decisions. Preparing for those eventualities is essential for everyone's peace of mind. You can help your partner focus on these concerns by presenting the following options, which you both may wish to discuss further with an attorney.

The Living Will

A living will is a directive to the physician regarding your partner's feelings about the use of life-support equipment or other extraordinary measures to sustain life. Because medical science has made it possible for humans to be kept alive by technology for an indefinite amount of time, many people are now choosing the right to die rather than be sustained in this manner. The result is the living will, now recognized as a legal document in all states.

However, it should be noted that the use of living wills is still not widespread. It is estimated that only about 15 percent of Americans across the country have signed living wills. Many doctors are not yet comfortable discussing what they view as a disturbing subject, and therefore do not suggest or encourage their patients to set up such a directive. In addition, because the legality of living wills is still being challenged, decisions are made—by the family or the doctor—that countermand the patient's wishes in about 25 percent of all cases.

For these reasons your partner may choose to appoint you (or someone else close to him or her) as a health care proxy—a person who is legally designated to make decisions about treatment and medical care—should your partner become impaired. Another option is to sign a *durable power of attorney for health care* to a person whom your partner trusts to uphold his or her wishes. A durable power of attorney allows someone to make legal and binding decisions about the way health care is administered should your partner become unable to make such decisions him- or herself.

If you and your partner decide to create a living will

and/or assign a health care proxy or durable attorney for health care, it is wise for you to do so with the aid of a lawyer. If your state has a living-will law, the form your partner must sign is printed in the state law. You may obtain a copy of the living-will form valid in your state from a law library or from an attorney. If your state does not have a living-will law, your partner may write his or her own living will. Your partner must sign and date any living will in the presence of two adult witnesses.

It's wise for your partner to place a copy of the living will and other legal documents in a safe-deposit box, to inform medical personnel and another responsible party of their existence, and also to make sure that his or her lawyer has a key to the safe-deposit box.

Advance Directive to a Physician

Unlike the generality of the living will, an advance directive to a physician provides specific instructions relating to your partner's particular case. Such a document helps absolve the physician from liability and minimizes his or her fear of a malpractice suit.

Last Will and Testament

Everybody needs a will, no matter his or her age or state of health. A will is simply a legal document stating an individual's wish for the settlement of his or her estate after death. A will is the best way to (a) determine the distribution of personal belongings and assets; (b) provide for family needs, including naming a guardian for minor children; (c) plan wisely for taxes, helping heirs minimize estate and income tax on what they in-

herit; and (d) make charitable contributions. Only by
having a will can one be sure that his or her wishes will
be carried out after he or she dies.

Being confronted with a serious illness may trigger
you and your partner to create or reevaluate a last will
and testament. To be sure that the document is valid,
you need the help of a lawyer and, depending on the
value of your partner's assets, a financial adviser such as
an accountant or bank trust officer.

Make sure that your partner updates all legal documents on a regular basis. A power of attorney or a
living will is only as good as a person's or institution's
willingness to accept it. Remind your partner to rewrite
important directives (if only by changing the effective
date) at least every two years.

TELLING FAMILY AND FRIENDS

Both the physical and the emotional issues related to
cancer may make it all too easy for both you and your
partner to withdraw from the world. Sometimes, it
might be the lingering social stigma of the disease itself,
other times, it could be the physical limitations the disease and its treatment pose, that makes your partner
hide the condition from friends and family. If that kind
of withdrawal occurs at first, stepping back out into the
world may be one of the toughest things the two of you
face.

Nevertheless it is essential that both you and your
partner find loving support from other people and that
you do so as soon as possible. The more you try to

protect the people who love your partner from knowing about the illness, the more you risk incurring their resentment and hurt feelings—and the farther away they will grow from both of you.

Will friends disappear, unable to handle the harsh reality or the frightening uncertainty of the illness? Perhaps. Even close families and stable relationships can be threatened by the pressures of a long-term illness. Emotional and physical exhaustion, frustration, and constant worry and care can all take their toll. But friendships built on solid foundations of respect and mutual interests will most likely flourish in the face of a new challenge.

Keep in mind that you all may be suffering from the same feelings of inadequacy, the same burdens of guilt, the same quiet anguish, the same sheer tedium of a prolonged illness. No one can or should be blamed or criticized for the ways he or she responds to the crisis of cancer or the threat of change or loss. Instead try to keep the lines of communication open and work together to fight the cancer that has threatened someone you love.

Tips for Telling People About Cancer

If you and/or your partner feel awkward or uncomfortable talking about the illness, the following hints may help:

• Decide with your partner whom to tell and when to tell them.
• Timing is important. If you wait too long, people

may feel betrayed by your secretiveness. On the other hand it may be best to wait until you have both gained some perspective about the diagnosis and have some idea of what the treatment plan will entail. That way you're more likely to feel in control and able to answer any questions your family and friends may have.

• Decide whom you and your partner need to tell personally. Talking about the illness can be tiresome and emotionally exhausting for both of you. Once you bring a close friend or relative into your confidence, ask him or her to tell those people in your family circle that don't need to hear the news directly from you.

• Try to anticipate how the person will react. You're better off not being caught completely off guard by a negative or fearful reaction, which may only upset you even more.

• Think about what you want or need from the person you tell. A shoulder to cry on? Help with caregiver responsibilities? State your needs as clearly as you can; it will help guide friends, relatives, and coworkers toward a positive reaction.

• Guide people to sources of information. Friends may not want to burden you with questions or may be too confused or worried to ask. Bring educational materials—pamphlets, brochures, or photocopies of research material—about the type of cancer your partner has that may help explain his or her situation more clearly than you may be able to do.

• When telling young children about a parent or other relative who has cancer, approach the matter as simply and with as many facts as possible. Even kids as young as three or four years of age are capable of understanding information about cancer if it is told to them in a simple, informative manner. Children have a remarkable power of imagination, and what they imagine is often far more devastating and difficult for them to handle than the actual facts.

It is important to give the child a chance to ask questions, not only at the time you tell him or her, but throughout the course of the illness. Children may be particularly afraid of things you may not think they're old enough even to consider, such as whether cancer is contagious or inherited. They should feel free to ask whatever is on their mind without being afraid of embarrassing or upsetting you or your partner.

Try to keep in mind that children will pass through many of the same stages of acceptance that you and your partner will, though maybe not at exactly the same time. They may become angry at your partner for being ill, or feel guilty for being well while your partner is sick. In fact it is common for young children to think that they are actually responsible for the adults in their lives getting sick—perhaps they wished them ill in a moment of anger—and it is important that you help them open up to you and discuss their secret fears and worries.

Finding Support

In addition to your family, friends, and coworkers, there are millions of people out there who know just what you're feeling. They want to help you deal with the many problems you face, and they can do it with firsthand knowledge that even the best health care professionals lack. They are your fellow cancer fighters and their partners, and they form a warm and loving network of support.

This year about 900,000 Americans will be diagnosed with cancer, and more than 3 million are still alive after an earlier diagnosis. Many of these people and their families belong to one of the hundreds of cancer support groups located in cities and towns throughout the country.

Most of these support groups are organized with the help of local hospitals and are linked to the American Cancer Society. Support groups meet on a regular basis, usually once a month, to discuss common problems, form friendships, and learn coping strategies from both professional guest speakers and fellow cancer fighters. Take advantage of this important resource by contacting your local American Cancer Society office.

As suggested at the beginning of this chapter, the very first step you, as your partner's primary caregiver, should take is to educate yourself about the type of cancer your partner has and the treatment alternatives suggested by his or her primary physician. Chapters 3 and 4 will outline the basic facts about cancer and cancer treatment for you and your partner.

THREE

Understanding Cancer

"When Allison came home and told me that her dermatologist found a strange-looking bump on her shoulder called a basal-cell carcinoma," recalls Phyllis, Allison's sister and roommate, "we both sort of brushed it aside. It wasn't serious, the doctor was going to simply scrape it away [in a procedure known as electrosurgery] in a couple of days. There wouldn't even be much of a scar. All Allison had to do was keep a close eye on the rest of her skin to make sure she didn't get another one."

According to Phyllis, the two sisters went on about their lives, barely giving a thought to what had just occurred. "Then about a month later, sort of out of the blue," confesses Phyllis, "it hit us both that Allison had had cancer. Granted, it was the most common and the least serious, but still it was cancer. We both wanted to know what it really meant. What was cancer, anyway? Why did my sister's body suddenly start to turn against itself?"

WHAT IS CANCER?

In the disease we know of as cancer, a cell—the smallest unit of living matter in the body—becomes corrupted and begins to grow abnormally. This corruption can occur spontaneously, through some internal malfunction within the cell itself, or it can occur when the cell comes into contact with an external agent that triggers a disruption of the cell's normal activity. Cancer, by definition, is a group of cells that multiply uncontrollably, resulting in a growth of malignant cells called a tumor.

Normally, every cell in the body "knows" how often and under what circumstances it is to reproduce and at what rate it will be destroyed or lost in the body. This information is part of the cell's genetic code. Indeed, most cells have a finite lifespan and are replaced at death in an orderly fashion. Some cells, like those of the skin and gastrointestinal tract, die and are replaced at a rather rapid rate. Other cells, such as liver and brain cells, live longer and are replaced much more slowly.

If cells are triggered by a cancer-causing agent or otherwise malfunction, this means that their genetic code is fundamentally altered. In effect, cancer cells lack the control to stop their growth processes and therefore continue to divide without internal restraint. At the same time, cancer cells do not die at a normal rate—in fact, they die only if they outgrow their blood supply—and thus continue to grow until they form a tumor.

There are two basic types of tumors: benign tumors and malignant tumors. Benign tumors are not cancer, they are growths composed of cells that very closely resemble normal tissue and tend to form a rounded mass. These cells, like healthy cells, are not inclined to invade other cells or tissues. Occasionally, benign tumors may cause problems in the body, such as when they press against a vital organ and need to be surgically removed. In most cases, however, benign growths require no treatment at all.

Malignant tumors, on the other hand, grow in a far more deviant manner. Unlike normal cells, malignant cells tend to spread to adjacent areas and invade normal tissues and organs. If cancer cells in the liver, for instance, grow unchecked, the growth formed will eventually crowd out and destroy healthy liver cells and prevent the liver from functioning properly.

All cancers begin with the corruption of a single cell. When that cell divides, there are two cancer cells; when they both divide, four cancer cells exist, and so on. Different cancer cells divide at various rates. The time it takes for a particular cancer to double its size is called its "doubling time." Fast-growing cancer may double in size over one to four weeks; slow-growing cancers may double in over two to six months. In fact, it may take a slow-growing cancer up to five years to double. When a tumor is large enough to be seen on an X ray, it usually has to be about one half inch (1 cm) in diameter. At this size it will contain about a billion cells. Until a malignant tumor has disrupted the function of a vital cell or otherwise produces symptoms, the person whose cells have gone awry may have no idea that he or she is ill.

In addition to encroaching on the healthy tissue from which it arises, some cancer cells may travel from the original site to another part of the body. When these cells invade distant tissue, it is called metastasis. The ability of cancer cells to metastasize is what makes cancer potentially deadly.

The Meaning of Metastasis

Some cancer cells may escape from the original, or primary, tumor and travel usually by one of three routes to different sites, where they may form new tumors. The three routes by which cancerous cells travel include

• *By local extension.* As the primary tumor grows, it may invade adjacent organs and tissues, forming roots that grow into the layers of surrounding tissue like a crab sticking its claws into the sand. Indeed, cancer was named for the Greek word for "crab"—*karkinoma*—by Hippocrates, the ancient Greek physician who compared a cancerous tumor to the hard center and claw-like projections of the crustacean.

• *Through the bloodstream.* Like other tissues of the body, a malignant tumor is fed nutrients and oxygen brought by blood vessels; arteries pump blood into the tumor, and veins take it away. Single cancer cells can escape through blood vessel walls, enter the blood-stream, and, if able to evade immune system cells that could destroy them, circulate through the body until they attach themselves to one or more organs at distant sites.

• *Through the lymph system.* The lymphatic system is composed of vessels that carry a liquid called lymph throughout the body. Lymph bathes the cells of the body and serves as a filter for impurities. Lymph contains immune-system cells that capture and destroy foreign cells, including viruses and bacteria. In addition to the vessels themselves, there are several lymphatic organs, including lymph nodes and the spleen. One of the most common ways for cancer cells to metastasize is by traveling through this vessel system. That is why the lymph nodes closest to the primary tumor are checked for evidence of cancer cells during the metastatic workup.

It is important to understand that all cancer cells are not alike and do not metastasize by the same route. A colon-cancer cell, for instance, looks and behaves differently than a cancer cell that originates in the liver. This remains true even after colon-cancer cells have broken away from the original tumor, traveled through the bloodstream or lymph system, and attached themselves to liver cells to form a tumor there.

Indeed, cancer is not one disease; it is many. In fact there are more than two hundred different types of cancer, similar to one another in that they are all characterized by the uncontrolled growth and spread of abnormal cells—cells that have been corrupted by as yet largely unknown agents. They are different because each type of cancer arises from a different type of tissue, behaves in a distinct way, responds to different kinds of treatment, and has a different prognosis.

WHAT CAUSES CANCER?

The short answer to the above question is "We still don't know," but the whole truth is far more positive and complex. Indeed the past few decades of cancer research have uncovered many clues about how and why this disease occurs in the body. Every day medical scientists come closer to identifying the agents that corrupt the first cell and how they are able to do so.

Cancer-causing Genes

One of the most exciting avenues of current cancer research concerns the discovery of oncogenes, genes that have lost their control mechanism or which have been triggered by certain agents to transform a healthy cell into a cancer cell. To date, scientists have isolated and identified dozens of different oncogenes in several kinds of cancer, including those of the bladder, breast, colon, and lung. Other kinds of cancer, including retinoblastoma, a rare and often fatal eye cancer, apparently occur when suppressor genes are missing from the genetic code.

Although some cancers have strong genetic components (if both parents lack the retinoblastoma-suppressor gene, for instance, their child is almost certain to develop the disease), most are caused when several "hits" by different triggers—not just the inheritance of a chromosomal abnormality—occur together. In fact it appears that cancer is at least a two-stage process and requires two or more "hits" by different triggers for an oncogene to "turn on" and stimulate the creation of a cancer cell.

The Cancer Triggers

Scientists have identified a number of corrupting agents that may lead to the development of cancer in susceptible individuals. Included among them are the following:

• *Viruses.* It has long been suspected that viruses—tiny disease-causing organisms—play a role in some cancers. It appears, however, that viruses do not act alone in producing cancer; not everyone exposed to a cancer-related virus develops cancer.

• *Carcinogens.* Scientists estimate that as many as 80 to 90 percent of all cancers may be related to substances in the environment we call carcinogens. The best-known carcinogen is tobacco and tobacco smoke, which is linked to the most common deadly cancer in the United States today: lung cancer. Exposure to radioactive material (including overexposure to X rays) has been known to cause cancer, as have industrial agents or toxic substances such as asbestos, coal-tar products, benzene, cadmium, uranium, and nickel.

• *Dietary influences.* Eating patterns may strongly affect the risk of developing cancer. Indeed, eating a healthy, nutritious diet may help reduce an individual's cancer risk by as much as 30 percent. Some things we consume appear to promote cancer development, including dietary fat, excessive alcohol, and food additives. Others, such as antioxidant vitamins and minerals such as C, E, and beta carotene, as well as dietary fiber, help prevent it.

• *Ultraviolet radiation.* Sunlight and other sources of ultraviolet light (such as tanning booths) are the leading cause of skin cancer, the most common cancer in the United States.

• *Hormones.* There is much evidence to support the theory that the development of some cancers in both women and men are related to the amount of sex hormones individuals are exposed to in their lifetime. Many cases of breast cancer and endometrial cancer are related to how much estrogen—the primary female hormone—the organ is exposed to during a woman's lifetime. Men, too, appear to be affected by hormonal levels; prostate cancer is far less likely to develop in men who have had their testicles removed before puberty and thus do not produce the male hormone testosterone.

• *Weaknesses in the immune system.* Researchers now believe that many cancerous cells are intercepted and destroyed by the immune system before they form tumors. The immune system, comprised of special cells that circulate in the blood and lymph, is our body's chief defense system. If the immune system is somehow weakened, however, such interceptions are not made and cancerous cells are allowed to live and reproduce. In addition recent research points to the possibility that the cancer cells themselves may release a potent molecule into the bloodstream that cripples the immune system, thereby allowing the cancer to take hold and spread. (More about the immune system and cancer treatment in Chapter 4.)

Unfortunately there are very few instances in which the exact cause of a specific cancer can be identified. Even lung cancer, which is directly linked to cigarette smoking in most people's minds, may be caused by another unknown factor: Not everyone who smokes develops lung cancer, nor has everyone with lung cancer smoked cigarettes.

There is only one reason for you to gain an understanding of the possible causes of your partner's cancer, and it is not so that you can find something—harmful genes, destructive environmental agents, or bad habits —to blame for your partner's disease. Indeed such a task is impossible; there are simply too many factors involved to pin the blame on any one of them. Instead learning how cancer begins will help you better understand why the therapies the physician recommends may work to destroy or undermine cancerous cells.

CLASSIFYING AND STAGING MALIGNANCIES

When your partner's physician talks about your partner's cancer, it is important that you understand the terms used to define and describe the disease. First, cancers are classified according to the type of cell and the organ from which they arise; there are four different types of cancer.

Carcinoma, the most common kind of cancer, arises in the epithelium, the layers of cells covering the body's surface or lining internal organs and various glands. The six most common cancers in the United States today—cancers of the breast, colon-rectum, female repro-

ductive system, lung, prostate, and skin—are all carcinomas and comprise nearly half of all cancers
diagnosed in any given year.

Carcinomas tend to increase in incidence with age.
The reason may be related to the fact that epithelial
cells are by nature the ones most frequently and persis-
tently exposed to the external physical, chemical, and
viral agents that are known to trigger cell mutations.

Sarcomas originate in the supporting (or connective)
tissues of the body, such as bones, muscles, tendons,
nerves, and blood vessels. Since supporting or connective tissue is found throughout the body, sarcomas can
be found anywhere in the body. If a blood vessel in the
liver develops a tumor, for instance, it is still a sarcoma,
even though it is found in the liver.

Leukemias begin in the blood-forming tissues—the
bone marrow, the lymph nodes, and the spleen. These
cancers are named after the type of blood cell that is
affected.

Lymphomas develop in the cells of the lymph system.
One specific kind of lymphoma is called Hodgkin's disease; all others are referred to as non-Hodgkin's lymphomas.

In addition to determining the type of cancer your
partner has developed, the pathologist (the specialist in
identifying cancer cells) can judge how fast the tumor
may grow by examining under a microscope cancer
cells taken from the tumor itself. A *well-differentiated
tumor* has cells that look very much like the normal
tissue they came from. A normal liver cell, for instance,
has a characteristic look. When a pathologist examines

cells from a well-differentiated liver tumor, he or she can see that it is a liver cell even if it is a cancer cell.

If a tumor cell is *undifferentiated,* on the other hand, it does not particularly look like the normal tissue from which it arises. Looking at a piece of undifferentiated tissue under the microscope, the pathologist may not be able to tell where the tissue was taken from. Undifferentiated tumors tend to be more aggressive than their well-differentiated counterparts. They usually grow faster, may spread earlier, and have a worse prognosis.

Another classification system used primarily to classify sarcomas and brain tumors refers to tumors as *high grade* or *low grade.* A high-grade tumor is immature, undifferentiated, and fast growing. A low-grade tumor is usually well-differentiated and slower growing. The pathologist will also examine the degree of necrosis (cell death) in the tumor as well as the status of the blood supply.

Armed with information about the type and behavior of your partner's particular cancer, your partner's physician will then begin what is called the staging process. Staging provides a standardized, concise summary of which tissues and organs the tumor has invaded or metastasized by applying a common and uniformly agreed-upon set of criteria to individual cases of cancer.

You and your partner should not be alarmed if several days to two weeks are devoted to the staging of your partner's cancer. While time-consuming and sometimes uncomfortable, the procedures used to stage cancer—biopsies, laboratory tests, and X rays—are essential to determining the prognosis and ultimately the treatment for your partner's cancer. Staging may occur before surgery is performed to remove the tumor, after surgery, or at both times.

The staging process involves finding the answers to the following three questions:

- How large is the tumor? (This question is usually answered before surgery.)
- Have cancer cells invaded nearby lymph nodes?
- Has the tumor metastasized and to which location?

Let's take these questions one by one so that you can gain an understanding of what your partner's physician is searching for with the many diagnostic tests he or she has prescribed:

- *What size is the tumor?* This information is derived with the aid of X rays and other imaging techniques and/or exploratory surgery.
- *Have tumor cells invaded nearby lymph nodes?* As you may remember, the lymph system is the primary route by which cancer cells travel through the body. If cancer cells in lymph nodes close to the original tumor are found, the lymph nodes are usually removed along with the tumor.
- *Has the tumor metastasized?* The final and most important piece of the diagnostic process consists of finding out whether or not cancerous cells have broken away from the primary tumor and found their way to one or more part or parts of the body. More than any other single factor, metastasis determines the type and level of treatment a cancer requires.

Once you and your partner have learned all you can about the type of cancer involved and the stage it is in, you and the health care team will meet to discuss the treatment options most likely to help your partner fight his or her cancer. Chapter 4 outlines the basic therapies currently available.

FOUR

Exploring Treatment Options

Fifty-year-old Martin Swann found out he had colon cancer after a routine rectal exam during his annual physical. His physician felt a lump in his lower colon and immediately ordered a series of diagnostic tests, including blood tests, urinalysis, and a colonoscopy, an examination of his colon with a special flexible tube fitted with a lighted microscope.

"I'm not sure how many tests he had, or what they were, it all happened so fast," recalls his wife, Sara. "Within just a week we were called into his doctor's office and told Martin had rectal-colon cancer. He'd need an operation and probably chemotherapy. But first they wanted to use radiation to see if they could shrink the tumor before they operated."

Sara was frightened, first about whether her husband would survive, then about what life would be like for them both after the colostomy, which would remove part of the colon and create an artificial opening through his abdomen.

"I knew, though, that I had to put aside the big fears and deal with all the things that would come before.

How did radiation work? How dangerous would the surgery be? Was there any way to avoid a permanent colostomy? When would chemotherapy start and how bad would the side effects be? I decided to get real practical, so I brought a notebook to our next doctor's appointments and asked every question about therapy I could think of."

Armed with those answers, as well as the information and advice of a consulting physician from whom they received a second opinion, Martin and Sara sat down together and sorted out the information and options before them.

"Although in the end we went with the treatment plan our first physician had recommended," Sara admitted, "we felt we were part of the team, so to speak, because we took the time to learn about what would be happening. We weren't so overwhelmed, and we didn't feel bullied. We were scared, but we were prepared."

As discussed in Chapter 1, one of your main tasks as a primary caregiver is to gather information and present options to your partner. In the last chapter you learned the ABCs of cancer—what may cause it and how it spreads, and how a physician evaluates individual cancer cases in order to determine appropriate treatment. This chapter brings you to the next step—understanding the treatment options to treat different types of cancer, including what treatment might work best for your partner's particular type and stage of cancer. It must be noted that treatment for cancer is highly individualized, so highly individualized in fact that any attempt in a book of this type to recommend any specific treatment plans would be meaningless and irresponsible. You and your partner will gather information from many sources, including both your physicians, other health care professionals, as well as an outside source such as the National Cancer Institute's Cancer Information Service (see "Appendix 1: Resources"), before making any decisions about cancer treatment. Even friends and acquaintances who have been treated for cancer can provide you with valuable advice.

YOUR PARTNER'S RIGHT TO DECIDE

At this crucial stage, when decisions regarding treatment are about to be made, it is important that you help your partner become an active member of the decision-making team, along with his or her physician and other health care professionals. Taking a positive, active role is far more apt to make your partner feel confident about the future than would remaining passive—even if he or she decides to follow every recommendation set forth by the physicians. Indeed you should stress to your partner that taking an activist role does not necessarily mean butting heads with the health care team, but offers instead an opportunity to exert as much control as possible in what may be a frightening situation.

Every state requires by law that your partner understand and accept any medical treatment being offered before it is administered. This legal standard, known as informed consent, has been in effect since 1957, when a federal court ruled that doctors are required to disclose to the patient "any facts that are necessary to form the basis of an intelligent consent by the patient to the proposed treatment." The necessary facts include information about the reasons for and associated risks and benefits of the treatment and about any alternatives that may exist.

Informed consent is required before anesthesia is administered, before most non-invasive tests and treatments, and before surgery. It is also required before a patient's participation in any investigational study or experiment (see below).

Before your partner consents to the suggested treatment plan, make sure that the following requirements are met to the best of your and your partner's physician's abilities:

• All relevant information is provided to you and your partner about the nature and purpose of any procedure or therapy, its risks and benefits, and any alternatives—including the alternative of no treatment—with their associated risks and benefits.

• Your partner understands the information offered. Talking it through with him or her is one way to make sure you both have a thorough grasp of the situation.

• Your partner gives his or her consent voluntarily, without feeling pressured or coerced by anyone, including you or any member of the health care team. Because your partner may feel overwhelmed, you as the primary caregiver should help your partner to take the time and exert the energy required to make a rational decision about his or her health care options.

DEFINING THE GOALS OF CANCER THERAPY

Once your partner's cancer has been diagnosed and staged, the physician is able to form a prognosis—a prediction or forecast of the probable course of the disease. In other words the doctor is able to make a highly informed judgment about your partner's cancer, based on the results of diagnostic tests, his or her own past experience, and a statistical analysis of others who have had the same disease.

In the not-so-distant past the prognosis for most advanced cases of cancer was very poor. In the 1930s about 25 percent of all those stricken by cancer in the United States were treated and survived more than five years after diagnosis. Even as recently as 1955 the future looked grim for most cancer patients; only 33 percent achieved long-term (five or more years) survival. Today, however, advances both in our understanding of the disease itself and in treatment modalities has increased the odds considerably: Well over 50 percent of all cancer patients remain disease-free for five years or more after receiving treatment. Although this statistic is just an average—the cure rate for some cancers, such as most skin cancers, is much higher than other more serious malignancies, such as liver or lung cancer—it points to the progress made in conquering this disease.

Indeed even cancer patients with very advanced cancers may benefit greatly from currently available therapy, adding either years to their life or quality to the time they have remaining to them, or both. Treatment therefore can have one or more basic goals:

• *Cure.* Cure is the goal for a wide range of cancers today; as stated above, over half of newly diagnosed cancer patients will be cured of their disease. The word *cure*, when used in discussing cancer, means that the disease has been in remission—no signs or symptoms of the disease remain—for a long enough period to indicate that the cancer has been completely destroyed.

In most cases a person treated for cancer is considered "cured" if the cancer does not recur within five years of completion of treatment, but the length of remission necessary differs from cancer to cancer. Many cases of skin cancer, for instance, are considered cured as soon as the tumor is removed; other types of cancer may remain in remission for up to ten years. Thus that length of time must pass without a recurrence for a cure to be assumed.

• *Long-term management.* Some stubborn, difficult-to-cure cancers can be controlled successfully over a period of several years, even a decade or longer with current therapy. Long-term management requires ongoing treatment to slow the growth and spread of cancerous cells while reducing or eliminating symptoms. Certain types of breast cancer, as well as some leukemias and lymphomas are the most common types of cancers considered chronic, although any disease that recurs but is responsive to treatment can benefit from long-term management.

• *Symptom relief.* Palliative treatment—treatment intended only to bring symptomatic relief to the patient—should be considered in cancer cases in which neither cure nor containment of the disease is possible. Palliative treatment may be considered an option for people whose cancer is discovered at an advanced stage, when the tumor has already become too large or spread too extensively to be removed by surgery or respond to other treatment, or is attached to vital organs. Pain management, medications for anxiety and depression, and other forms of symptom relief are included in the treatment plan.

In discussing a comprehensive plan with your partner and the health care team, keep in mind that the treatment goals may change as the treatment phase continues. For instance if a particular cancer does not respond to drugs chosen or if cancer cells are resistant, long-term management rather than cure becomes the goal; he or she will require long-term ongoing observation and treatment to keep the disease in check. If a cancer becomes more aggressive and resistant to therapy, palliative treatment may become the most feasible option in cases where cure and/or long-term management was once considered possible.

On the more optimistic side, any number of cancer patients thought to have "incurable" cancers have been able to fight and win the battle against the disease with the help of doctors, medical therapy, and their own fierce will. Obtaining the most accurate diagnosis, understanding the risks, benefits, and alternatives of any treatment plan offered, and receiving treatment as soon as possible remain the best ways of achieving a successful result.

UNDERSTANDING RISKS AND BENEFITS OF TREATMENT

As discussed, cancer treatment is highly individualized; each and every cancer patient faces unique challenges and has different physical and psychological strengths to help meet them. In developing your partner's individual treatment plan, the physician will take several factors into consideration:

• *The stage of the cancer.* As discussed in Chapter 3, the results of diagnostic tests and procedures performed tell the physician the physical qualities of your partner's particular cancer: the type and size of the tumor, how the tumor behaves, and if and where cancer cells have spread.

• *Your partner's age and general state of health.* Fighting cancer takes a great deal of stamina and both physical and emotional strength. If your partner is ill with another condition, particularly one that is itself life-threatening or debilitating, aggressive anticancer therapy may be counterproductive or even more dangerous than no treatment at all. Likewise if your partner is of an advanced age and is thus nearing the end of his or her life, the time gained by treating the cancer may be outweighed by the unwelcome side effects of aggressive therapy.

• *Quality of life with and after treatment.* Treatment for advanced cancer often produces painful, disfiguring, and disabling side effects without necessarily providing any guarantee that the cancer will be cured. Some cancer fighters may choose a less aggressive therapy in order to live out their remaining time with as much health and energy as possible.

Again, just as the goal of treatment may change during the course of therapy, so, too, may the balance of risks and benefits; a side effect once considered endurable may become unacceptable if the treatment does not succeed in eradicating or reducing the cancer. Both you and your partner should remain informed about the progress of treatment and be willing to revise your expectations and goals along the way.

STANDARD CANCER TREATMENTS

In 1971 the United States Congress passed the National Cancer Act, a landmark piece of legislation that put the fight against cancer on the national and international agenda for the first time. The act appropriated funds for cancer research and empowered the National Cancer Institute—a federal institution—to coordinate research and treatment programs and to give support to investigators and physicians throughout the nation.

Since that time the search for the cause and cure of cancer has advanced by leaps and bounds. Not only have the standard treatments of cancer—surgery, radiation, and chemotherapy—greatly improved, but new techniques have been fostered that have already helped many people on an experimental basis and hold great promise for cancer patients in the very near future.

Short descriptions of each type of treatment and how you, as a primary caregiver, can help your partner prepare for them, are given below. It should be noted that most patients' treatment is "multimodal." This means that many different forms of therapy may be used, either one by one or in combination. For example if the cancer is found to be inoperable, either radiation and/or chemotherapy may be used. If all the cancer is removed by surgery, then with some types of cancer "adjuvant" therapy (chemotherapy, radiation, or both) may be used to kill any remaining cancer cells.

Surgery

Surgery is the oldest and remains the most effective form of cancer treatment. Indeed more cures are achieved by surgery than by any other form of therapy. If your partner has cancer, there is a very good chance that he or she will see a surgeon at some point during the course of treatment.

Your partner's primary physician may recommend surgery under a variety of circumstances:

• *As a diagnostic tool.* Surgery is used to excise tissue for biopsies as well as to allow the physician to visually examine a tumor within the body.

• *To remove the cancer.* For many types of cancer, surgery holds out the best prospect for a cure. For this to be possible the tumor must be contained in an area of the body from which it can be safely removed. Sometimes, radiation or chemotherapy will be administered before surgery to shrink the tumor and thus make it more operable.

• *To remove metastases or recurrent tumors.* Even

after the primary tumor has been eradicated, a cancer patient may require surgery to remove cancer cells from other parts of the body or if cancer returns to the original site.

• *To relieve symptoms.* Surgery remains a primary form of palliative treatment, used to remove tumors that are causing pain, bleeding, or other symptoms—even if the cancer cannot be cured.

• *To reconstruct or rehabilitate.* Removing a tumor from the body may cause disfigurement (as in the case of breast cancer) or functional problems, and surgery is often used to reconstruct the appearance of the body and to restore function.

No matter why your partner undergoes surgery, it is important to understand that it is a serious procedure, involving risks that must be weighed against the benefits. Patients with severe heart/lung disease, for instance, may have a heart attack or stop breathing during surgery. Anesthesia in itself may be risky, especially if your partner is of an advanced age or has other physical problems, particularly heart or lung disease. It is important that your partner discuss these and all risks of surgery with the physician prior to the procedure.

Helping Your Partner Cope with Surgery

• Find the most qualified surgeon by discussing credentials with the oncologist and making sure that the surgeon is board-certified by the American College of Surgeons.

• Make sure that your partner is as physically fit and

healthy as possible. If he or she smokes, try to get him or her to stop as soon as possible after the decision to perform surgery is made. Lung and breathing problems are the most common complications following surgery; clearing the lungs—even if only for a few days—will significantly reduce the risks of your partner developing these complications.

• Know what to expect following surgery, from waking up from general anesthesia to caring for wounds and scars to undergoing physical therapy. The more you and your partner understand about the postoperative period, the better prepared you will both be. Read Chapter 6 for tips on how to help your partner recuperate.

Radiation Therapy

Radiation therapy is the second most common form of cancer treatment, after surgery. About half of all people with cancer will need radiation treatments at some point during their therapy. Most commonly, it is used to reduce the size of a tumor before surgery or to destroy any remaining cancer cells after surgery. Radiation therapy is also used to treat patients with advanced cancer who require symptom relief—the radiation will be used to shrink local areas of the cancer that are causing pain or other symptoms. Radiation cannot be used to eradicate cancers that have spread to distant parts of the body.

Radiation may be delivered in two different ways— external and internal. In *external-beam radiation,* a machine sends X rays or gamma rays into the tumor. In *internal radiation,* a radioactive substance such as radium is put into the body by means of surgical insertion of a sealed container. Which method is used depends on many factors, including the type of tumor involved and the risk of side effects.

The key to successful treatment with radiation is getting the right amount of radiation to the tumor without harming healthy tissue in the process. A physician trained to use radiation to treat cancer, called a radiation oncologist, will work with the primary physician to design a treatment program that will send a predetermined dose to the right area in the most efficient way possible.

Radiation treatments may damage healthy tissue and thus result in unpleasant side effects, including fatigue, nausea and vomiting, skin rashes, and more localized problems. If radiotherapy is administered to the neck area, for instance, healthy mouth and gum tissue may become irritated and sore, making it difficult for the cancer patient to chew and swallow. Radiation used to treat brain cancers may destroy hair follicles, causing the cancer patients to lose his or her hair in that area.

It is important to note that not everyone who undergoes radiation develops side effects; in fact, the majority of cancer patients experience only minor discomfort or none at all.

External beam radiation is usually given daily five days a week, continuing from two to eight weeks on an outpatient basis. Using multiple treatments of radiation, instead of one massive dose, helps give normal cells the chance to recover from contact with radiation and therefore reduce the risk of side effects and/or reduce their severity.

Internal radiation, on the other hand, usually requires hospitalization. Depending on the type of device used, tiny radioactive seeds are placed inside the body at the site of the cancer. Cancer patients are kept in a hospital during this treatment, which may last anywhere from one to seven days. Because the implant is radioactive, patients are isolated during this period.

Helping Your Partner Cope with Radiation Therapy

• Before your partner receives radiation, make sure you both know all the facts. Ask for help in weighing the risks and benefits of radiation for your partner's particular type and location of cancer. Some points to cover with the radiation oncologist include: What dose of radiation your partner will receive, length of treatment, kind of radiation, and the success rate the treatment has had in other patients.

• Make sure that your partner receives radiation from a board-certified radiation oncologist (a physician who has received three or more years of formal training in the use of radiation to treat cancer and has passed an examination in this area). Check with your partner's primary physician or look in the American Medical Association's Directory of Physicians at your local library.

• Think in practical terms about the demands treatment may make on your partner's energy and your time. Many patients become exhausted with radiation and need help in getting to and from the hospital for treatments. Child care may become an issue if hospital-

ization is required. Thinking ahead will save stress on
you both.

• Read Chapter 6 for tips on how to deal with common side effects of radiation therapy.

Chemotherapy

The term chemotherapy means treatment of cancer
with drugs. Taken either orally or through injection,
chemotherapeutic agents are used to treat a wide variety
of cancers. They may be given alone or in combination
with surgery or radiation or both.

Although a single drug may be used in some cases,
patients are usually given a combination of different
drugs. Indeed the form of treatment and combination of
drugs used vary enormously with each type of cancer.
Some treatment plans involve a regular stay in the hospital over a period of weeks, while others are done on
an outpatient basis.

Chemotherapy is an established way of destroying
hard-to-detect cancer cells that have spread and are circulating through the body. In fact, of the three basic
cancer treatments, chemotherapy is the only one able to
combat cancer's most lethal weapon—the ability to metastasize or spread through the body. Chemotherapy
has the advantage of traveling in the bloodstream to
almost all parts of the body and thus is able to eradicate
cancer cells that are out of reach of the scalpel or radiation beam. It is also used to provide long-term control
for some cancers and to relieve symptoms in patients
with advanced cancer.

Chemotherapeutic agents are available by mouth in

tablet form, by intramuscular injection, and by intravenous drip. Newer methods of delivery include implanted infusion ports (catheters implanted beneath the skin so that repeated injections are not necessary) and ambulatory pumps (portable devices connected to implanted catheters that deliver chemotherapy on a continuous basis), among many others.

The length of treatment with chemotherapy is equally variable. Some cancers achieve cure or remission within six months to a year; other, more stubborn malignancies or cancers the doctors feel will recur, may be treated with chemotherapy for an indefinite period.

Chemotherapy drugs are cytotoxic, which means that they may be poisonous not only to cancerous cells but to healthy tissue as well. This explains why some cancer patients develop unpleasant side effects from chemotherapy, including hair loss, nausea and vomiting, rash, infections, and bleeding.

Helping Your Partner Cope with Chemotherapy

• Remind your partner that anxiety over treatment and treatment side effects may actually worsen the reactions. A more relaxed attitude toward chemotherapy—which you can help him or her to assume by learning as much as possible—may lead to fewer bad experiences.

• Like radiotherapy, chemotherapy may cause exhaustion and nausea. You may need to arrange to be with your partner in the hours following treatment in order to provide comfort and care when he or she needs it most.

• Read Chapter 6 for tips on how to treat specific side effects of chemotherapy.

Biological Therapy

Biological therapy attempts to use the cancer fighter's own immune system to eliminate cancer cells. As you may remember from Chapter 3, the immune system is designed to recognize and destroy any foreign substance found in the body. Until recently, however, it appeared that the immune system could not recognize cancer cells as foreign, perhaps because there are so few differences between normal and tumor cells. Biological therapy attempts to strengthen the immune system and improve its ability to destroy cancer cells.

Although almost all biological therapy remains under investigation, in some kinds of cancer it has become accepted treatment. Generally speaking, biological therapy consists mainly of treating the immune system with highly purified proteins—complex compounds made up of amino acids—that help activate the system or help it do its job more effectively. These proteins are injected into the bloodstream.

Experimental Therapies

Every day cancer researchers come closer to finding a cure to this disease. Although the ultimate goal has not yet been achieved, enormous progress has been made in finding more effective treatments that have fewer side effects than standard therapies. Among the new avenues in cancer treatment are these:

Hyperthermia is the use of heat to help destroy tumors. In certain cases heat applied to the tumor for about an hour once or twice a week has shown promising results when used in combination with radiation and/or chemotherapy. Hyperthermia has been used in this way to effectively treat advanced primary breast cancer, melanoma (a type of skin cancer), certain types of cervical cancer, and advanced tumors involving lymph nodes containing metastatic cancer.

Bone marrow transplantation involves replacing defective bone marrow with healthy bone marrow. Bone marrow contains immature blood cells, including those that will develop into red cells, white cells, and platelets. The procedure may be used in some cases of several types of cancer, especially leukemias for patients with chronic myelogenic leukemia. It may also be used in cases where high dosages of chemotherapy and/or radiation necessary to kill cancer cells also destroy the bone marrow. Without a bone marrow transplant these patients would soon succumb to infections and other serious consequences of a lack of healthy, mature blood cells.

It must be noted that bone marrow transplantation is a dangerous procedure with many risks to the patient, including increased risk of infection, bleeding, and graft vs. host disease (rejection), and as such is still considered experimental as a cancer treatment in most cases. With help and advice from the health care team, you and your partner should carefully weigh all of the risks and benefits before agreeing to the operation.

Laser therapy involves the use of high-intensity light to destroy tumor cells. Although the technique is now used mainly to relieve serious complications, such as bleeding or obstruction, advances in laser techniques may make this mode of therapy more effective and reliable in the future.

CLINICAL TRIALS AND INVESTIGATIONS

Depending on the type and stage of your partner's cancer, the oncologist may recommend a new kind of treatment, such as one of the experimental therapies described above or, more commonly, a new drug or drug combination. Studies of experimental therapies, also known as investigational or clinical trials, may be right for your partner if his or her cancer is unlikely to benefit from standard treatment options.

Before any new drug, device, or procedure is released for general use, it must be tested on humans. Most clinical trials are designed to improve the best standard treatment for a particular cancer. It takes the results of treatment on several hundred and sometimes several thousand patients to prove the effectiveness of certain drugs or procedures.

Before any clinical trial can be conducted, it must be approved by a human-use committee, which is made up of physicians and other health care personnel who have no connection to the study being considered. Such a review board has two main tasks: First, to ensure that the anticipated benefit is commensurate with the potential risk to the patient. Second, to determine that the patient is fully informed about the study before consenting to participate. The consent form itself must be complete and comprehensible, as discussed at the beginning of this chapter.

Many cancer patients have benefited from participating in a clinical trial; indeed almost every advance in cancer treatment over twenty years has come about through this process. However, your partner should carefully consider the risks and benefits as they relate to his or her specific cancer before agreeing to undergo experimental therapy. Some of the questions your partner should ask include the following:

- What will happen if I have the standard treatment instead of this treatment?
- What are the risks and side effects of the treatment? Will the treatment make me sicker?
- Can I stop treatment at any time?

If the answers to these questions are acceptable to your partner, then he or she should ask for the consent form designed for this particular study. It will further explain and delineate the details of the process. Your partner should read it carefully—and have his or her physician read it as well—before signing.

COMPLEMENTARY THERAPIES

One further note about cancer treatments: In addition to the standard and investigation therapies currently available, there are myriad unproven "cures"—substances or procedures that claim to work miracles without the scientific data to back them up. To people with cancer and their families unproven treatments advertised in such a way can look very appealing, especially when no conventional treatment is known to be effective. You and your partner should resist the lure of these elixirs, however, making sure never to leave conventional treatment for an unproven method without first discussing the matter with the primary physician and other certified health professionals.

On the other hand there are several other established "alternative" or "complementary" treatments that may very well help to alleviate the symptoms and side effects of cancer. When they are used in conjunction with standard therapies, most physicians agree that they are legitimate therapeutic approaches. Such methods include the following:

• *Acupuncture.* An ancient Chinese form of medicine, acupuncture is based on the philosophy that a cycle of energy flowing through the body controls health and that pain and disease develop when there is a disturbance in the flow. To remedy this, acupuncturists insert long, thin needles at specific points along meridians, or longitudinal lines flowing through the body. Each point influences a different part of the body. Many cancer patients use acupuncture to help relieve pain from symptoms or side effects of drugs.

• *Homeopathy.* Homeopathy means "like disease" and as such attempts to treat symptoms with substances that are likely to produce a similar set of symptoms. Homeopaths prescribe minute quantities of a substance similar to, but not identical to, the causative agent of the disease.

• *Foods that fight cancer.* Nutrition therapy should never be used as a replacement for conventional medical treatment following a cancer diagnosis, but there is some early research to indicate that certain foods can retard the spread of cancer cells. Studies show that foods high in beta carotene (dark-yellow and green vegetables and fruits); fish rich in omega-3 fatty acids (the fattier fish, including salmon, mackerel, and bluefish); and garlic, especially when eaten raw, all have anticancer properties. And for women with breast cancer, eating a diet rich in cruciferous vegetables (broccoli, cauliflower, brussels sprouts) and wheat bran may reduce circulating estrogens, which are thought to promote cancer spread.

• *Mental healing.* In the past the psychological aspects of cancer were often neglected. Today, however, mainstream medicine has come to accept the fact that attitudes and emotions may well have an effect on health, in both positive and negative ways. In Chapter 7 you'll find out how you can help your partner tap into the most positive and healing aspects of his or her mind and body while reducing negative influences such as stress and anger. (See also "Techniques for Fostering the Mind-Body Connection on page 167.)

As you've discovered, the options your partner has available to treat his or her cancer are many. As discussed at the beginning of this chapter, it is important to remember that no decision about treatment is irrevocable. You should both feel free to evaluate the progress of therapy with the physician on a regular basis and if necessary redesign the treatment plan to more effectively fight the cancer.

In Chapter 5 you'll learn about the six most common cancers in the United States today. You'll find out how these cancers may develop, how they are treated, and some of the challenges these specific cancers pose to the cancer fighter and his or her caregiver.

FIVE

Meeting the Enemy: The Six Most Common Cancers

As mentioned in Chapter 3, there are more than two hundred different types of cancer. However, the majority of people with cancer in the United States suffer from one of six different types: skin cancer, lung cancer, colo-rectal cancers, breast cancer, prostate cancer, and female-reproductive, or gynecological, cancers. Together these six diseases account for well over half of all cancers diagnosed each year.

It is likely, then, that your partner has been diagnosed with one of these six cancers. In this chapter you'll discover just a few of the most pressing challenges your partner now faces and learn how you both can work together to meet them. Even if your partner suffers from another type of cancer, you may want to read through this chapter for the insights into cancer care that can be applied in general ways.

Understand, however, that you will need to work in close consultation with your partner's physician and other members of the health care team to understand and cope with the wide range of concerns posed by these complicated diseases. This book is limited in the details it can provide about the many coping techniques available to you and your partner.

BREAST CANCER

Breast cancer is the most frequently occurring cancer in women. Current statistics confirm that 1 out of 9 American women will develop breast cancer in her lifetime. (Breast cancer rarely occurs in men.) About 182,000 women will develop breast cancer in 1996 and about 46,000 will die from it. Breast cancer is most common in women over the age of fifty, although about one-third of all cases occur in women thirty-nine to forty-nine years old, and it also occurs, rarely, in younger women.

Breast cancer is one of the more curable cancers—when diagnosed and treated in its earliest stages. About 90 percent of localized breast cancer is now cured, compared with about 50 to 70 percent of more advanced cases. Periodic, regular screening of healthy women—beginning when they are thirty to forty years old—with physical exams and mammography has resulted in more and more women surviving breast cancer every day.

Frequently breast cancer is discovered by the woman herself, or her sexual partner, who finds a lump or thickening in the breast tissue. The majority of lumps are benign growths, but the most effective way to tell is to remove a small amount of tissue—either through surgery or a technique known as needle aspiration—from the lump and send it to the laboratory for examination, a procedure called a biopsy.

Causes/risk factors: The specific causes of breast cancer in each individual are usually unknown, although hereditary factors, diet (especially one high in fat), and menstrual and pregnancy history may all play some role in the development of this cancer.

Types: There are several different kinds of breast cancer distinguished mostly by their rates of growth and tendency to spread to other parts of the body. Breast cancer usually spreads by way of the lymph system, starting with the axillary lymph nodes, located in the armpit, or in lymph nodes under the sternum.

Treatment overview: Surgery remains the first-line treatment for breast tumors. In brief there are three different surgical options available to women with breast cancer depending on the extent of the disease. Until the last twenty years or so most breast cancers were treated by *radical mastectomy,* which involved removing the entire breast, axillary lymph nodes, and the chest muscles. Today, even if the breast tumor is large and has spread to axillary nodes, another surgical procedure is performed, called the modified radical mastectomy.

In a *modified radical mastectomy* the tumor and axillary nodes are removed, but the pectoral muscles are not. If the cancer is small enough, the surgeon may remove only a portion of the breast in an operation called a quadrantectomy, which removes a smaller part of tissue along with the tumor and lymph nodes. The lymph nodes are removed to provide information about the risk of recurrence and metastasis and to better define the need for other treatment methods.

The least radical and disfiguring of breast cancer surgeries, the *lumpectomy* involves the removal of only the breast lump with a small margin of surrounding tissue. A slightly more invasive surgery is the *segmental mastectomy,* in which the lump plus a larger wedge of normal tissue is removed. Recent studies point to the effectiveness of lumpectomies; preliminary results of a National Cancer Institute study show that the less-disfiguring lumpectomies, when followed by radiation, are as effective as removal of the entire breast in women with early-stage breast cancer. You and your partner should understand these surgical options and discuss how they apply to your partner's cancer before surgery is performed.

After surgery most women will receive additional (adjuvant) therapy to prevent the cancer from returning or to ensure that any errant cancer cells have been destroyed. Adjuvant therapy may consist of radiotherapy, chemotherapy, hormone therapy, or some combination of these techniques. The type of recommended therapy often depends on whether the woman has gone through menopause, whether there was any cancer found in the lymph glands at the time of surgery, and the biologic characteristics of the cancer.

In addition to the standard treatments, several experimental techniques are currently under investigation for advanced cases of breast cancer. The use of bone marrow transplantation for metastatic and high-risk early-stage breast cancer is being studied. This type of bone marrow transplantation, which uses the patient's own marrow, appears to produce better response rates than conventional therapy in cases of advanced metastatic disease. Treatment with monoclonal antibodies is also under investigation.

Deciding on the Treatment Plan

The first challenge for most women with breast cancer and their partners is to decide on an appropriate treatment plan, including what type of surgery she and her physician choose to perform in order to remove the tumor, as well as adjuvant therapy. The decision is especially difficult for breast cancer because of the potentially disfiguring aspects of the surgery necessary to remove the tumor.

What You Can Do to Help

• Gather as much information as possible about the treatment options available and present them to your partner. This means talking with physicians and other health care personnel, reading books such as this one that help you better understand breast cancer, and using resources like the National Cancer Institute's Cancer Information Service.

• Support your partner's decision about treatment and work with her physician to make her recovery as easy as possible. If your partner requires a mastectomy, ensure that she discusses breast reconstruction options with her physician before the surgery.

Recuperation After Surgery

If your partner has a mastectomy, she will require several weeks of physical recuperation following the operation. Her chest and arm will usually feel numb and sore, and the incision will need special care. The less radical the surgery, of course, the less time is required for recuperation.

What You Can Do to Help

• Learn to care for the wound, which will take about a month to six weeks to heal fully. (A lumpectomy incision takes about two weeks to heal.) See "Wounds and Scars" in Chapter 6, "Treating Symptoms and Side Effects: An A-to-Z Guide."

• Within a day or so of the surgery your partner should begin to perform deep-breathing exercises to help expand the chest wall. You can assist by counting aloud from 1 to 5 as your partner inhales and counting down from 5 to 1 as she exhales. If you use a soothing voice and encourage her along the way, the task may seem less painful.

• As soon as the doctor gives his or her okay, your partner should begin to exercise her arm. One exercise involves squeezing a tennis ball or a rolled-up pair of socks with the hand on the affected side of the body. This will help your partner gain strength in her arm. To help her gain full mobility of her arm, her physician or physical therapist may suggest that she stand about six inches from and facing a wall, bending her elbows and placing both hands on the wall. Then, slowly, she should work both her hands up the wall until she feels a pull or stretch on the affected side. You can help by marking in pencil her progress up the wall over a period of several weeks.

• If your partner has a lumpectomy, the recovery period from the surgery itself will be much less intense.

However, the radiation and/or chemotherapy that usually accompanies this surgery may cause its own side effects. See Chapter 6 for more information.

Breast Reconstruction

Breast reconstruction is a surgical procedure for mastectomy patients that rebuilds the breast contour and, if the woman desires, the nipple and/or areola. Almost any woman can have breast reconstruction, regardless of her age, the type of surgery initially performed, or the number of years since the operation.

If your partner's cancer is small and shows no signs of having spread to axillary lymph nodes, it may be possible for reconstruction to be performed immediately following the mastectomy, therefore alleviating the need for a second operation. With larger cancers, however, breast reconstruction takes place several weeks or even months later, especially if radiation and chemotherapy are used along with surgery.

There are several different types of breast reconstruction, and your partner, her physician, and a board-certified plastic surgeon—preferably someone with experience helping breast cancer patients—must work together to decide which one is right.

What You Can Do to Help

• Gather information and present options—preferably before your partner's surgery takes place.
• Make sure that your partner continues to receive careful follow-up care from her primary physician.

Breast reconstruction will not hide a recurrence of breast cancer, but it won't prevent it either, and your partner must remain alert.

• Support your partner if she decides *not* to have breast reconstruction. Some women, especially those who must go through several different surgical procedures as well as chemotherapy and radiation to treat their cancers, choose not to undergo another operation.

Issues of Self-esteem and Sexuality

Sexual problems have been linked to mastectomy more often than to any other cancer treatment. The sexual problems faced by women who have, or have had, breast cancer stem from both physical and psychological sources. In our culture we are taught to view breasts as part of beauty and femininity. If a breast is removed, it can leave a woman insecure about her attractiveness and her partner's sexual feelings toward her. In addition the breasts and nipples are also sources of physical sexual pleasure; breast stimulation adds to sexual excitement for many women.

After any surgery for breast cancer the breast area will feel and look different. With a lumpectomy the breast may be scarred or have a different shape or size. With a mastectomy the whole breast is gone, including the nipple which is a sensitive sexual organ—at least until and unless reconstruction is performed. Chemotherapy and radiation each cause their own set of side effects that can interfere with sexual pleasure. It may take time and special understanding from her partner for a woman to adjust to these changes.

What You Can Do to Help

• If your partner feels less attractive after surgery, try to help her rebuild her self-esteem. Remind her, first, that feeling attractive is only one aspect of her self-image. Even if she does not feel attractive at this time, she should remember all of the other parts of her self—her sense of humor, her professional accomplishments, her spiritual strength—that make her the unique person she is. Later, when she's ready, you can help her concentrate on the physical aspects of her beauty once again.

• If you are her sexual partner as well as her primary caregiver, you must be as open and honest as possible about your own feelings. It is perfectly normal for you to feel awkward or even a little frightened when you first resume sexual relations. There are many techniques for getting past this stage—spending time simply touching each other's bodies without attempting intercourse is one proven method—and you and your partner should not hesitate to get some counseling from the primary physician or a licensed sex therapist.

• Read the "Sexual Problems" entry in Chapter 6 for more tips on how to make your sex life more satisfying for you both.

COLO-RECTAL CANCER

Cancer of the large bowel, which includes the colon and rectum, is the third most common type of cancer. About 150,000 new cases are diagnosed and approximately 61,000 people die from colo-rectal cancer every year. Colo-rectal cancers affect men and women in equal numbers and comprise 15 percent of all cancers in the United States. Taken together, they are second only to lung cancer as a cause of cancer deaths in the United States.

Colo-rectal cancer is highly curable when detected and treated in an early stage; unfortunately many people delay seeking medical attention even when they experience symptoms. Most cases of colo-rectal cancer are discovered by a physician during a routine rectal examination and/or chemical testing for blood in a stool sample. When symptoms do occur, they include a change in bowel habits (change in frequency, shape, or size of stools), blood in the stool, and/or having the urge to defecate when there is no need.

Types: Most colo-rectal cancers develop in the glands of the inner lining of the mucosa and are called adenocarcinomas.

Causes/risk factors: Colon cancer commonly occurs in people with a family history of the disease, a personal or family history of polyps (benign growths) in the colon or rectum, and ulcerative colitis and other colon disorders. In addition most epidemiologists associate colo-rectal cancer with diet—in particular, the low-fiber, high-protein, high-fat-content diet that characterizes the eating habits of most Americans today.

Treatment overview: Surgery is the primary treatment for colo-rectal cancers, resulting in the cure of about 50 percent of all cases. Tumors should be removed whenever practical—even if there is metastasis—because complications such as the blockage of the bowel or bleeding might otherwise develop. The standard surgery removes the portion of the bowel with the tumor along with the entire lymph and blood vessels that feed the area. In most cases the bowel can be reconnected. However, the procedure may require the creation of a colostomy—an artificial opening in the abdomen for elimination of body wastes. The colostomy may be temporary, to give the colon a chance to heal, or permanent if the lower part of the rectum has to be removed.

Adjuvant chemotherapy and/or radiotherapy decreases the risk of recurrence and increases the chance of long-term survival; this is especially true when the two adjuvant therapies are combined.

Handling Side Effects of Surgery and Radiation

After treatment for any type of cancer, your partner will require special attention to treat the side effects of surgery, radiation, and chemotherapy. Surgery to remove colon or rectal cancer usually involves a hospital stay of about eight days and recuperation time at home of several weeks, with a gradual reintroduction of normal activity. Radiation and chemotherapy may cause, in some but not all patients, several unpleasant side effects.

What You Can Do to Help

• Read Chapter 6, "Treating Symptoms and Side Effects: An A-to-Z Guide," for tips on how to make hospitalization more pleasant, how to care for wounds and scars, and how to care for a host of other problems your partner may face.

Care of Stomas

In about 15 to 20 percent of all cases of colo-rectal cancer, a permanent colostomy—the creation of an artificial opening in the abdominal wall—is necessary. In many other cases of colo-rectal cancers, a temporary colostomy is required to allow a part of the bowel to heal after surgery. After the area is healed (a process that may take from several weeks to several months), the opening—called a stoma—is closed and the bowel is reconnected so that the normal elimination process can continue.

If your partner requires a colostomy, the stoma, or ostomy, created will require special care. If that care is taken, your partner should be able to live a full, normal, and healthy life. Although the specifics of ostomy care go far beyond the scope of this book, there are several excellent resources for you and your partner to seek out.

What You Can Do to Help

• Make an appointment for you and your partner to meet with an enterostomal therapy nurse (an expert in the care of ostomies), preferably before the surgery takes place. He or she will be able to help prepare you both for the changes that come with a stoma.

• Basic care for the stoma include washing the area gently every day with warm water, making sure the pouch is emptied when it is one-third full, and changing the pouch at least once or twice a day. Your partner's diet and exercise habits should not have to change once the healing process is over. Further information about the care that your partner's specific type of stoma requires will be provided by the primary physician and enterostomal therapy nurse.

• For further help in coping with the physical and emotional side effects of a stoma, contact the United Ostomy Association (see "Appendix 1: Resources") to arrange for an ostomy visitor to meet with you and your partner. The visitor is a person who, like your partner, has had colostomy surgery and is thus uniquely qualified to help you both cope with your new day-to-day challenges.

The United Ostomy Association, in conjunction with the American Cancer Society, also conducts support groups throughout the country that allow ostomates (people with ostomies) and their families to share their feelings and concerns in a friendly, compassionate environment.

Sexual Concerns

Unlike surgeries to treat many female and male reproductive system cancers and bladder cancer, colostomy surgery *does not* interrupt or damage the neural pathways that excite and maintain sexual arousal. Nor, with proper care, should a colostomy pouch interfere with normal intercourse. With love and patience you and your partner should be able to return to your normal sex life as soon as your partner has recovered from surgery and any adjuvant-therapy side effects. Keep in mind, however, that both you and your partner may initially feel awkward about the changes that have taken place.

What You Can Do to Help

• Be patient with yourself and your partner. It may take you both some time to get over the trauma of the cancer diagnosis and treatment, and even more time to adjust to the stoma.

• There are many practical tips that may help you both better enjoy sexual intercourse. For instance, to minimize rubbing against the appliance, you and your partner should choose positions for sexual activity that keep your partner's weight off the ostomy. Placing a small pillow over the ostomy faceplate may help if your partner enjoys the bottom position during intercourse. Talk to an enterostomal nurse or an ostomy visitor for other suggestions.

• Read the "Sexual Problems" entry in Chapter 6 for more information.

GYNECOLOGICAL CANCERS

Cancer of the female reproductive organs was once one of the most common causes of cancer death among women but, thanks to new screening techniques, the incidence has declined dramatically in recent years. Today, there about 75,000 cases of cancer of the cervix, the ovary, and the uterus (specifically the uterine lining or the endometrium). About 13,500 cases of invasive cervical cancer occur each year, 34,000 cases of endometrial cancer, and about 21,000 cases of ovarian cancer; overall, about 15,000 women die of a gynecological cancer every year.

Cervical Cancer

Over 90 percent of cervical cancers are called squamous cell carcinomas because they start in the surface cells lining the cervix. (About 5 to 9 percent start in the glandular tissue and are thus called adenocarcinoma.)

Causes/risk factors: The risk of cervical cancer is increased by a history of viral genital infections, such as genital warts and herpes, as well as having multiple sex partners.

Treatment overview: Today, most cases of cervical cancer are caught in an early stage and can be cured by minor surgery to remove cancerous cells of the cervix. In more advanced stages radiation is added to the treatment plan, but this may cause atrophy of the upper vagina and vaginal scarring. If the cancer has invaded adjacent tissue and is recurrent, surgical removal of the rectum and/or bladder and the cervix, uterus, and vagina may be necessary. Chemotherapy is being investigated for women at high risk for recurrent disease as well as used concurrently with radiation in women with large cancers.

Ovarian Cancer

The most common form of ovarian cancer, known as epithelial carcinoma, arises from the cells on the surface of the ovary. Epithelial carcinoma of the ovary is further divided into five major types—undifferentiated, clear cell, edometroid, mucinous, serous—and each of these types is further divided into grades, according to how aggressive they appear upon microscopic examination. Other, rarer kinds of ovarian cancer are germ-cell tumors, which arise from the eggs, and ovarian stromal tumors, which arise from supportive tissue.

Causes/risk factors: Ovarian cancer, which will develop in one in every seventy American women, usually occurs in postmenopausal women. Women who have never had children appear to be at greater risk for developing ovarian cancer than those who have been pregnant and given birth. There may also be a genetic disposition to this cancer in rare cases.

Treatment overview: In women with early-stage cancer, one or both ovaries are usually removed (with or without the removal of the uterus). In advanced cancer surgical removal of as much of the tumor as possible, as well as the removal of the uterus, both fallopian tubes, both ovaries, and as much of the visible cancer as possible is attempted. In most cases chemotherapy is begun from one to two weeks after surgery and continued every three to four weeks for at least six cycles. Radiation therapy may be helpful for patients with early stages of ovarian cancer who have no visible cancer remaining after their operation.

Uterine Cancer

Endometrial cancer—carcinoma of the lining of the uterus—arises from the glands of the lining of the uterus. There are several subtypes of this disease, including adenocarcinoma, which accounts for about 90 percent of all endometrial cancers.

Causes/risk factors: Endometrial cancer is linked most directly to the amount of estrogen the uterus is exposed to over a woman's lifetime; it is seen mostly in older women between the ages of fifty and sixty-four with a history of infertility, late menopause, obesity, and prolonged estrogen therapy after menopause. The drug Tamoxifen, used to prevent recurrence of breast cancer, also increases risk of endometrial cancer.

Treatment overview: The standard therapy for most cases of endometrial cancer involves the removal of both fallopian tubes and ovaries and, if cancer is present, removal of pelvic lymph nodes as well. Depending on the stage of the cancer when it is diagnosed, radiation therapy applied to the pelvic area is often added two to six weeks after surgery.

Although each type of gynecologic cancer has its own set of causes and prognoses, they all have similar symptoms and side effects.

Sexual Dysfunction

Although most women—an estimated 95 percent—who undergo treatment for gynecological cancer eventually regain their former sexual patterns, there may be both physical and emotional hurdles that you and your partner must face together. Surgery required to treat the cancer may change the shape of the vagina, radiation may irritate the entire pelvic area, and chemotherapy may exhaust and nauseate your partner. Your partner may feel "less of a woman" due to the loss of her female reproductive organs; some of these feelings are psychological, but many are physical, especially if treatment causes her to have premature menopause. The loss of fertility can weigh heavily on your partner's mind—and your own—if you had planned to have children before cancer developed.

What You Can Do to Help

• Some physical symptoms are easily alleviated. Vaginal dryness caused by chemotherapy and radiation, for instance, can be treated with vaginal lubricants such as K-Y jelly. Estrogen therapy may be available to your partner who has had her ovaries removed if her cancer was not estrogen-receptor positive.

• If your partner continues to find intercourse painful, encourage her to speak with her physician. Corrective plastic surgery may be necessary to remove excess scar tissue. Sessions with a sex therapist may help you and your partner find alternative ways of attaining sexual pleasure if vaginal intercourse is difficult or painful.

Side Effects of Surgery and Treatment

Chemotherapy, radiation, and hormone therapy are often used as primary or adjuvant treatment for gynecological cancers. As your partner's primary caregiver, you should be aware of the possible symptoms and side effects these treatments may cause and how they can be eased.

What You Can Do to Help

• Talk to your partner's physician and other members of the health care team about what your partner should expect in terms of side effects, preferably before treatment begins.

• Read Chapter 6, "Treating Symptoms and Side Effects: An A-to-Z Guide," for information about treating common problems.

LUNG CANCER

Lung cancer is the most common form of cancer seen in the United States (apart from skin cancer), accounting for about 172,000 new cases of cancer every year. Today it remains the most deadly cancer for both women and men. Indeed, as of 1985 the lung cancer death rate overtook the mortality for breast cancer in women, due in large part to the dramatic increase in women smokers during the past several decades.

The symptoms of lung cancer include a persistent cough, chest pain, and recurring pneumonia or bronchitis. Unfortunately by the time lung cancer is diagnosed, it is usually well advanced. The overall cure rate is low: Only about 9 percent of all patients survive five or more years.

Types: There are two main types of lung cancer, each with its own cellular abnormalities: small-cell lung cancer and nonsmall-cell lung cancer. Small-cell lung cancer, also known as oat-cell cancer, is the more aggressive of the two types, tending to spread quickly to distant parts of the body. Nonsmall-cell lung cancer, also called squamous cell carcinoma, does not spread to other parts of the body as rapidly, and generally is more easily treated.

Causes/risk factors: The majority of lung cancers are caused by smoking, and the risk of lung cancer increases in direct relation to the number of years someone smokes and the number of cigarettes smoked each day. Workers exposed to industrial substances such as asbestos, nickel, chromium, and other carcinogens are also at higher risk of developing lung cancer, especially if they also smoke cigarettes.

Treatment overview: The treatment plan for lung cancer depends on the specific cell type and whether the lung cancer has metastasized. Surgery is the most effective form of treatment for nonsmall-cell lung cancer. Unfortunately only a minority of persons with nonsmall-cell lung cancer can be helped by surgical treatment, because it is usually discovered after the cancer has metastasized. Surgery is rarely used to treat small-cell lung cancer at all, even if the cancer seems to be localized to the lung, because it is such an aggressive disease.

Chemotherapy and radiation are combined to treat most all types of lung cancer. Radiation is also used to treat metastasis to the brain, the most common site of lung cancer spread.

Respiratory Problems

It is likely that your partner's lung cancer will require surgery to remove some or all of one lung. Even if surgery is not required, your partner may have some difficulty breathing and suffer from periodic shortness of breath due to the damage the disease has done to his or her lungs. In addition many lung cancer patients have a concurrent lung disease, such as emphysema, that makes normal respiration difficult.

What You Can Do to Help

• If your partner has had surgery, encourage him or her to practice breathing exercises that will increase the efficiency of the lungs and the strength of the inspiratory (inhaling) muscles. There are several exercises that a physician and/or a respiratory therapist can help to teach your partner.

In the meantime talk your partner through the following routine, which may help strengthen the diaphragm, the muscle that separates the lungs from the abdominal cavity. Direct your partner to

1. Lie on his or her back with the head and neck supported by pillows.
2. Breathe in and out slowly in a rhythmic pattern and try to relax.
3. Put his or her fingertips of one hand on the abdomen, just below the base of the rib cage at the center of the chest. Inhale slowly and feel the diaphragm lift the hand.
4. Practice pushing the abdomen against the hand as the chest becomes filled with air. The chest itself should remain motionless.

5. Repeat the exercise, by inhaling slowly to the count of 3 and exhale while counting to 6.

Your partner should practice this exercise until he or she is able to take ten to fifteen consecutive breaths in one session without tiring.

• To help avoid infections, make sure your partner knows how to release the accumulation of secretions that may collect in the lungs with any chronic lung disease. One method is the controlled cough, in which a deep breath is taken, then held, then let out in two sharp coughs. After resting for a moment your partner should repeat this procedure, keeping a box of tissues close at hand in case the cough produces sputum.

The Possibility That Therapy May Not Be Successful

The prognosis for most cases of lung cancer remains poor, but every day new advances are being made. While you and your partner should try to be realistic about the likely outcome of his or her disease, you should never lose the optimism that is an integral part of the fight against cancer. Even if the cancer is terminal, there are ways you can work together to make the time that is left as physically painless and emotionally fulfilling as possible.

What You Can Do to Help

• Gather information about all aspects of your partner's particular type of lung cancer and what the prognosis may mean for the rest of your partner's life. Knowing the facts is a good way to alleviate anxiety.

• If necessary, talk to your partner's physician about finding a therapist with experience in dealing with cancer patients facing a poor prognosis. Join a support group for further aid.

• Read Chapter 9, "Coping with Death and Dying," for more information if the prognosis is poor.

PROSTATE CANCER

Each year approximately 280,000 men are diagnosed with prostate cancer in the United States, making it the third most common cancer among men, after skin cancer and lung cancer. Prostate cancer is seen mostly in older men, with an average age of seventy-three at the time of diagnosis.

Early prostate cancer usually develops without any symptoms. Therefore a rectal examination, in which a doctor inserts an index finger into the rectum to check the prostate for any unusual swelling or nodules, is an essential screening technique and diagnostic tool. In recent years, a screening test, called the prostate-specific antigen test or PSA, has become an effective diagnostic tool. This simple blood test should be performed in conjunction with a digital rectal exam. If there are symptoms at all, they may include difficulty in urination because the prostate encircles the uppermost part of the urethra, the tube that carries urine from the bladder for elimination. Any prostate enlargement will encroach on the urethra and thus obstruct the flow of urine. (It should be noted that the same symptom may be caused by a completely harmless condition called benign prostate hypertrophy, also common in older men.)

Types: Nearly all prostate cancer arises from the glands of the prostate; glandular cancer (adenocarcinoma) accounts for 95 percent of all prostate cancer cases. Other types stem from supporting or connective tissues or develop in the ducts within the prostate, but are quite rare.

Causes/risk factors: Apart from increasing with age, risk factors for the development of prostate cancer are unknown, although there is some speculation about the relationship between prostate cancer and industrial carcinogens. A high-fat diet may also be a factor. The risk of prostate cancer is twice as high in blacks than in whites and is lowest for Asians, for as yet unknown reasons.

Treatment overview: Treatment depends on the stage of the disease and whether there is evidence of spread to other organs. Patients with localized disease have a good chance of living out their normal life expectancy after the prostate gland is removed or the tumor is treated with radiation. The surgical approach, known as a radical prostatectomy, was previously associated with a risk for impotence because the pelvic nerves were severed during the operation. Fortunately a new procedure spares the nerves and leaves two thirds of its recipients potent. All patients who have their prostates removed, however, will be infertile, since the prostate produces the fluid that transports the sperm.

An alternative to surgery in early, localized prostate cancer involves the insertion of radioactive iodine seeds into the prostate—a method that results in impotence about 5 percent of the time. External radiation may be used, but it fails to control the disease in about one third of men and often results in impotence.

Advanced prostate cancer requires systemic treatment with both chemotherapy and hormone therapy. Since the cancer depends on the male hormone (testosterone) in 80 percent of cases, hormone manipulation often succeeds in halting the cancer. Removal of the testes (orchiectomy) accomplishes this task, as does administration of female hormones (estrogens) in pill form. When orchiectomy or hormonal therapy fail, chemotherapy may be used in advanced stages, but the results are generally poor.

Sexual Dysfunction

Although the risk of permanent impotence exists, the sexual problems that most men experience after cancer treatment are temporary. For instance pain with erection or ejaculation may well disappear soon after treatment is complete. The stress of treatment can also reduce hormone levels for a few weeks, causing decreased desire or problems with erection.

Unfortunately some cancer treatments may indeed permanently alter a man's sexual function. Men who have this surgery have "dry" orgasms, because the vessels that produce and deliver semen have been removed, making them infertile. Although the majority of men remain potent, some men never recover the ability to have erections after radical prostatectomy.

What You Can Do to Help

• Be patient. It may take some time—perhaps a few weeks or months—following treatment before your partner feels physically and emotionally ready to resume sexual relations. It may also take time to find out if any sexual dysfunction is medical or psychological in origin. Your compassion and love will go a long way toward making this transition an easier one for the cancer fighter in your life.

• If your partner can no longer have an erection, he may want to consider having a penile prosthesis implanted. Talk the possibility over together with his doctor.

• If you and your partner had intended to have children, discuss with your partner and his doctor whether or not it is possible—before surgery or radiation—to store some of his sperm for artificial insemination at some time in the future.

• Consider visiting a sex therapist. Any sexual problem can respond to counseling from a sex therapist. A therapist can help a man deal with the anxiety and fear that often comes with prostate cancer and cancer treatment as well as help couples adapt to permanent changes in function to have a fulfilling, exciting sex life.

• Read the "Sexual Problems" entry in Chapter 6 for more information.

Urinary Incontinence

Some men find that a protastectomy causes them to lose their ability to control urine. The muscular and neural systems that control the retention or release of urine are complex; not only may surgery and radiation cause permanent or temporary incontinence, but fatigue and long periods of bed rest may also have an effect as well. Fortunately, there are many treatment alternatives to help with this problem.

What You Can Do to Help

• Ask your partner's physician for advice. He or she may suggest specific exercises to strengthen the pelvic area, or bladder-training techniques to regain control of urination.

• Suggest that your partner make a few adjustments to his daily routine—altering medication schedules, urinating more often than usual, avoiding taking liquids for several hours before bedtime—to see if the problem is alleviated in any way.

• When incontinence cannot be eliminated, special aids can help. Absorbent undergarments are available that neutralize the odor of urine and keep the skin fairly dry. Devices can be used to catch the urine, such as a type of condom that fits over the penis and drains urine through a tube into a plastic bag. Discuss these and other aids with your partner's physician.

SKIN CANCERS

With more than 1.2 million new cases diagnosed every year, skin cancer is the most common form of cancer in the United States today. It is also the most treatable: More than 90 percent are curable with surgery. One in every three new cancers is a skin cancer, and it is estimated that 40 to 50 percent of fair-skinned people who live to be sixty-five years old will have at least one skin cancer.

Because it is almost always diagnosed early and rarely invades distant body parts, skin cancer is considered the least serious and most curable cancer. The most prevalent types of skin cancer—basal cell and squamous cell —are two to three times more common in men than in women and almost always easily curable. Melanoma, a much more serious and invasive cancer, is increasing yearly. In 1961 the number of Americans who died from malignant melanoma numbered just over 2,000; in 1991 that number had increased to more than 6,000. The American Cancer Society estimates that the number of expected deaths related to melanoma in 1995 will be about 7,200 men and women.

Types: Ninety percent of all skin cancers are one of two types of malignancies: basal cell and squamous cell carcinomas. These types of skin cancers tend to be quite localized and rarely metastasize. Melanoma, a still rare but increasingly more common form of skin cancer, is much more aggressive and is often fatal. Melanomas are usually black or dark skin lesions that can occur on any part of the body. The risk of spread depends on how large the tumor is and how deeply it has invaded underlying tissues.

Causes/risk factors: Skin cancers, including melanomas, are caused by sun exposure, especially in light-skinned, blue-eyed, and fair-haired individuals. With melanomas, however, intermittent episodes of intense sun exposure causing sunburns, rather than the long-term exposure associated with basal and squamous cell cancers, are the culprit. Melanoma is most common in people in their forties to sixties and is rare before puberty.

Treatment options: The treatment for both basal cell and squamous cell cancers is similar. The object is to remove the cancer completely but leave as much normal tissue as possible and thus minimize cosmetic side effects. Current treatments include electrosurgery (the use of an electric needle that burns the cancerous tissue), chemosurgery (the use of chemicals with traditional surgery), cryosurgery (the use of liquid nitrogen to freeze the cancer), and radiation. Any of these treatments can be curative in better than 90 percent of cases if the cancer is small. If it is large or in an area that is difficult to treat, cosmetic surgery following the removal of the cancerous tissue may be necessary.

For malignant melanoma, surgery to remove the tumor and a large margin of normal tissue is essential. A skin graft is often needed to cover the surgically created wound, which may be deep. If the cancer has spread to adjacent lymph nodes, several diagnostic tests—chest X rays and liver, bone, and brain scans—should be conducted to see if the cancer has metastasized. If other organs have been affected, chemotherapy may be effective (about 20 percent of people with metastases will improve), but the prognosis tends to be poor.

Coping with Scars

Fortunately current methods of removing small, localized basal and squamous cell carcinomas minimize scarring in patients with skin cancer. If your partner's tumor is large, however, the wound created by the surgery may require some cosmetic surgery to repair the damage.

What You Can Do to Help

• Work with your partner and the primary physician to find a qualified, board-certified plastic surgeon, preferably someone who has extensive experience treating wounds caused by surgery for skin cancer.
• Read the "Wounds and Scars" entry in Chapter 6 for tips on how to keep incisions clean and sterile during the healing period.

The Risk of Recurrence

Like all cancers, skin cancer has a tendency to recur. Fortunately, as long as the new tumors are detected and treated quickly, they pose no increased risk to the long-term survival or health of the cancer fighter.

What You Can Do to Help

• Skin cancer can appear anywhere on the body. You can help your partner catch a malignancy early by helping him or her examine the body very carefully, from head to toe, front and back, at least once a month.

• Encourage your partner to avoid long-term or intense exposure to the sun and to use high-protection sunscreens whenever he or she is outside.

Coping with Side Effects of Chemotherapy and Radiation

The treatment of malignant melanoma is often quite aggressive, and your partner may experience serious side effects.

What You Can Do to Help

• Read Chapter 6, "Treating Symptoms and Side Effects: An A-to-Z Guide," for more information about the general problems faced by chemotherapy and radiotherapy patients and their caregivers.

SIX

Treating Symptoms and Side Effects: An A-to-Z Guide

As you've learned from reading the last three chapters, cancer and the treatment necessary to cure or control it may cause a variety of symptoms and side effects. Some of them are painful and life-threatening, others merely annoying and uncomfortable. In either case you, as the primary caregiver, can help your partner cope with these physical effects of the disease.

At the same time, it is important to understand the power of positive thinking in helping you both cope during the critical phases of treatment, when symptoms and side effects are likely to be at their worst. As we'll discover further in Chapter 8, no one can say for certain how much of our general health is due to our state of mind. The same is true for the way we cope with chronic illness. If your partner can wake up looking forward to the day's events and activities—even the challenges—with hope and confidence, it's almost certain he or she will feel in better control of symptoms and side effects.

Neither you nor your partner should forget the power of a great big belly laugh. As hard as it may seem at times, try to find some humor in your situation and point out the funny, wonderful things in the world to your partner. Indeed laughter is the best medicine in the world, and it's something you and your partner can share.

In the meantime the A-to-Z Guide will help you and your partner monitor and control the symptoms and side effects of cancer and cancer treatment. Read through the entire guide or look through the list below to find the topic that most concerns you and your partner at this moment. Here is the list of topics, in alphabetical order:

Appetite, loss of	Infections
Blood in stool	Leg cramps
Blood in urine	Mouth sores
Confusion	Nausea and vomiting
Constipation	Pain management
Dehydration	Sexual problems
Diarrhea	Shortness of breath
Dry mouth	Skin sores
Dry skin	Sleep problems
Falls	Swallowing problems
Fatigue	Swelling
Fever	Weight gain
Hair loss	Wounds and scars

APPETITE, LOSS OF

Both the disease itself and the side effects of both chemotherapy and radiation treatment for cancer—to say nothing of the anxiety of being ill—may cause your partner to lose his or her appetite. Unfortunately appetite is lost just when the patient needs it most; studies show that cancer patients need hundreds more calories and at least twice the amount of protein as those people not fighting a life-threatening disease. As discussed in Chapter 4, both normal and cancerous cells can be destroyed by chemotherapy and radiation, and thus the normal cells that line the mouth, stomach, and intestines may be destroyed by chemotherapy.

Foods and liquids may thus taste different to your partner, who may then lose all desire to eat. In particular, sweet foods often lose much of their sweetness, and proteins begin to taste extremely bitter.

Other side effects of therapy, including nausea and difficulty swallowing, may contribute to this problem. A feeling of fullness in the stomach, even when little food has been consumed, is another typical symptom. Weight loss is often a result. Fortunately most cases of poor appetite due to treatment are temporary and are relieved a few weeks after the frequency or amount of chemotherapy and/or radiation decrease or are discontinued.

What You Can Do to Help

• Serve foods high in calories that are easily digestible (e.g., pudding, ice cream, milk shakes, eggnog).

• If protein tastes bitter to your partner, suggest that he or she salt food more than usual (cured meats such as ham, bacon, or sausage work well too). Marinating meats in fruit juices or soy sauce may also help improve the taste. Ask your physician, however, if he or she can use salt freely.

• Using plastic rather than metal utensils may also reduce the bitter taste of many foods.

• If your partner becomes nauseous at the smell of food, try serving food cold or at room temperature to decrease its smell and taste.

• Add a high-protein supplement to the diet (e.g., Ensure, Isocal, etc.) if the loss of appetite lasts for more than a few days.

• Try serving small, frequent meals instead of three larger meals.

• Your partner's appetite should improve in between doses of chemotherapy or radiation, so make sure he or she takes advantage of these periods by eating more food than usual.

• Create a relaxed, comfortable atmosphere at mealtimes—and make sure that mealtime is a family time too. That way your partner can feel part of the "real world" even if he or she is not feeling his or her best.

• Encourage your partner to eat as much as he or she can manage, but try not to nag—that will only increase anxiety, making it even more difficult to eat.

• Take a walk with your partner about an hour before a meal. Exercise will often stimulate the appetite.

Warning Signs!

Call the doctor if your partner

- Cannot eat for more than a day or two
- Loses five pounds or more
- Feels pain when eating
- Does not urinate for an entire day or does not move the bowels for more than two days
- Continues to feel nauseous for days and/or vomits for more than twenty-four hours following chemotherapy

BLOOD IN STOOL

Blood in the stool may be caused by a variety of conditions, including irritation of the anus during a bowel movement, after a prolonged bout of diarrhea, or after straining hard to expel feces. Hemorrhoids (blood vessels that extend beyond the anal area) are the most common cause, followed by ulcers in the bowel or anus. If your partner notices blood on toilet paper or in the toilet bowl after a bowel movement, or sees streaks of blood in the feces, it's important for you not to panic, but also essential that your partner see his or her doctor for an evaluation.

What You Can Do to Help

• Keep your partner calm. Blood in the stool is an alarming symptom but, as described above, it often has a benign cause.

• Suggest that your partner wash the anal area very carefully with warm soapy water, rinse well, and pat dry. If he or she is bed-bound and unable, perform this task yourself.

• If hemorrhoids are diagnosed, warm sitz baths are helpful in easing symptoms.

• Caution your partner not to strain bowel movements, or use enemas or laxatives. However, a stool softener can be quite helpful and soothing. Ask the doctor to recommend one.

Warning Signs!

Call the doctor immediately if your partner

• Notices blood on toilet tissue more than three times within a week
• Has black or dark red stools

BLOOD IN URINE

Also called hematuria, blood in the urine occurs when someone is bleeding in some part of his or her urinary system and the blood is being flushed out along with the urine. Several different kinds of chemotherapeutic drugs are known to irritate the bladder. After these drugs are broken down in the body, they are eliminated through the kidneys into the bladder. High concentrations of medicine in the urine may irritate the bladder walls, causing them to bleed. Urinary tract infections, injury to the urinary tract, or kidney or bladder stones are other common causes, which is why it is important to notify the physician as soon as possible. Many people with hematuria also experience difficulty urinating as well as low-back pain.

Hematuria tends to occur only when chemotherapy has been given for more than four or five years. Once it occurs, your partner's physician will attempt to change from one drug to another, less toxic one. After several weeks off the offending medication, the hematuria should subside.

What You Can Do to Help

• As long as the fluids are unrestricted, make sure your partner drinks at least two quarts of water or other fluids every day. This will help to flush out the medication from his or her urinary tract as quickly as possible.

• Remind your partner to urinate every night before going to bed to rid the body of toxins before a long sleep.

Warning Signs!

Call the doctor if and when your partner

- First sees blood in the urine or discoloration of the urine
- Feels pain upon urination
- Is unable to urinate or has high frequency of urination
- Has fever or chills

CONFUSION

Your partner may experience periods of confusion and loss of concentration for many different reasons connected to cancer and cancer treatment, including direct effects of the chemotherapy and radiation treatments on the brain, side effects from the medications used to treat nausea and vomiting, and the increased fatigue associated with the disease and its treatment. Both pain and drugs to treat pain are especially apt to cause a loss of concentration and confusion.

What You Can Do to Help

- First, you and your partner should discuss the problem with the physician. Often medications can be changed or diets supplemented to relieve the underlying causes of confusion, but it is up to the doctor to determine the appropriate therapy.
- Stay with your partner as much as possible when

he or she is feeling confused. Touch him or her often during conversation, and talk slowly and in short sentences so that he or she can understand you more easily.

• Keep a calendar and clock within your partner's view so that he or she can remain oriented to the date and time without having to ask.

• During periods when he or she is experiencing confusion or loss of concentration, assist your partner with washing, going to the bathroom, and in other daily tasks that may be difficult for him or her to perform alone. Make sure you make it clear exactly what you are doing and why so that he or she will feel comfortable and safe.

• Protect your partner from injury. Take over the cooking if your partner has periods of confusion, and put side rails on the bed if you feel he or she might get out of bed only to lose balance or not know where he or she is. Do not leave medications within reach of your partner when he or she is feeling confused.

Warning Signs!

Call your partner's doctor if and when

• Your partner becomes confused suddenly or if the confusion becomes worse
• If violence occurs during these periods of confusion

CONSTIPATION

Constipation is the infrequent or difficult passage of hard feces (stool), which often causes pain and discomfort. It is caused by too little fluid, and not enough exercise, in the bowel. Lack of activity, poor food and fluid intake, emotional stress, and general weakness can all contribute to this usually temporary problem. Chemotherapy drugs are often constipating, since they may diminish the nerve impulses to your intestine, thus preventing food from being moved through the digestive tract. Narcotics such as morphine and codeine, antidepressants, tranquilizers, sleeping pills, and many other types of medication also have disruptive effects on the digestive system.

By itself constipation is not a cause for concern. Contrary to popular belief, there is no medical necessity to move the bowels every day; the body does not become "poisoned" if defecation does not occur every day. However, if your partner becomes constipated, he or she may feel bloated and uncomfortable.

What You Can Do to Help

• Get advice from your partner's physician. He or she may recommend a mild laxative or an enema or change your partner's medication. Do not try to diagnose and treat the problem yourselves since there may be more to it than you realize.

• Encourage your partner to drink at least two quarts of water or other fluids every day. If your partner has difficulty eating, he or she should try to drink highly nutritional fluids (milk shakes and eggnogs, etc.) instead of plain water, since liquids can be filling and may further decrease appetite.

• Help your partner incorporate *daily* exercise into his or her life as soon as possible. Exercise stimulates the intestinal reflexes and helps restore normal elimination.

• Increase the amount of high-fiber foods in the daily diet, including bran and wheat germ, fresh raw fruits and vegetables with skins and seeds, and fruit juices. Avoid serving chocolate, eggs, and cheese, as these foods tend to exacerbate constipation.

• Avoid using over-the-counter laxatives, stool softeners, and enemas, unless recommended by your partner's physician.

Warning Signs!

Call the doctor if and when your partner

• Has not had a bowel movement in more than two days
• Has blood in or around area or in stool (also see page 114)
• Has persistent cramps or vomiting

DEHYDRATION

Dehydration is the loss of fluid from body tissues. Without enough fluid the body is unable to perform vital functions with efficiency. People with cancer may become dehydrated as a side effect of cancer therapy, particularly frequent vomiting and/or the inability to eat and drink enough food and fluids. The signs and symptoms of dehydration—which usually develop over a period of several days—are dryness of skin and mouth, decreased urine volume, and inability to swallow dry food.

What You Can Do to Help

• Provide your partner with plenty of different kinds of fluids—water, carbonated water, fruit juice, sodas, and so forth—and try serving them both iced and at room temperature.
• Apply lotion frequently to dry skin.
• Use ice chips to relieve dry mouth (see page 124 for more tips on good mouth care).
• If your partner is bed-bound, keep a small cooler filled with some favorite beverages on a nightstand so that he or she can sip liquids throughout the day.

Warning Signs!

Contact your partner's physician if and when

• Diarrhea or fever continues for more than twenty-four hours
• Your partner's urine is either very dark in color and of a small amount, or if there is no urine for twelve hours or more
• Your partner becomes disoriented, dizzy, or confused

DIARRHEA

Diarrhea is the passage of loose or watery stools three or more times a day with or without discomfort. In those with cancer, diarrhea occurs when healthy cells in the digestive tract are destroyed by chemotherapy or radiation, making it impossible for the water in the intestine to be properly reabsorbed back into the body. In addition to being a common side effect of chemotherapy and radiation, diarrhea may be caused by bacterial and viral infections; surgery; anxiety; supplemental feedings containing large amounts of vitamins, minerals, sugar, and electrolytes; and tumor growth. Diarrhea caused by chemotherapy or radiation therapy may continue for up to three weeks after treatment.

What You Can Do to Help

• Encourage your partner to drink plenty of fluids; contrary to popular belief, drinking more fluids will not cause more diarrhea. It is best that beverages be served at room temperature, since very hot or cold liquids will increase the tendency for the intestinal tract to contract, causing cramping. Try fruit juices and noncaffeinated beverages.

• Prepare foods high in protein, calories, and potassium but low in fiber. Good choices include cottage cheese, eggs, baked potato, boiled white rice, cooked cereals, macaroni, and smooth peanut butter.

• Avoid serving foods that typically cause gas or cramps, such as beer, beans, and spicy foods. Encourage your partner to eat slowly to avoid swallowing air with the food, which may also cause cramping.

• Try offering several small meals to your partner instead of three large ones.

• Add nutmeg to foods in order to slow down the movement of the intestine.

• Suggest to your partner that he or she clean the anal area with a mild soap after each bowel movement to protect it from developing sores. A layer of nonprescription ointment which contains xylocaine (a mild anesthetic) will soothe the anal area if it is sore.

Warning Signs!

Call your partner's physician if and when

- Your partner has diarrhea more than six times per day and there is blood in the stool
- Your partner loses five or more pounds after the diarrhea starts

DRY MOUTH

A lack of saliva is caused by chemotherapeutic drugs, radiation treatment to the mouth and neck, and many different kinds of medication to treat pain, stomach disorders, and infections.

In addition to causing discomfort, dry mouth is also unsanitary and potentially harmful to your partner's teeth and digestion. Saliva prepares the food for swallowing and begins the breakdown of food for absorption farther along the digestive tract. Saliva also contains immune substances that help to protect the teeth, gums, and soft tissues of the mouth from attack by bacteria and fungi. Bad breath is an unpleasant side effect of dry mouth, as are cracked lips and burning sensations of the gums and tongue. Other side effects include dried, flaky, whitish-colored saliva in and around the mouth or thick, mucousy saliva that stays attached to the lips when the mouth is opened.

What You Can Do to Help

• Frequent cleansing of the mouth and teeth is necessary to prevent mouth sores from developing. Purchase a soft-bristle toothbrush for your partner, and encourage him or her to brush every two to three hours.

• Encourage your partner to rinse his or her mouth every two hours with salted water (one teaspoon of salt to one quart of warm water). Avoid commercial mouthwashes, since they contain alcohol, which has a drying effect on the tissue lining of the mouth.

• Limit the amount of coffee, diet sodas, and liquor your partner drinks, for they can both dehydrate the body and irritate the mouth. Hot and spicy foods should also be avoided.

• Provide your partner with sugar-free candies or sugarless gum to suck on or chew, which help stimulate the production of saliva.

• Add liquids and lubricants to solid foods by using gravies, melted butter or margarine, yogurt, or mayonnaise.

• Cocoa butter and olive oil can soothe parched tissue if spread on the tongue and the inside of the mouth.

• Discuss the problem with your partner's physician, who may prescribe an artificial saliva if the problem cannot be resolved in other ways.

Warning Signs!

Contact your partner's physician if and when

• Your partner's mouth remains dry for more than three days
• Mouth sores develop

DRY SKIN

Chemotherapy and radiation treatments take their toll on the skin, causing it to become flaky, red, and sometimes sore. Dry skin is also usually related to dehydration (see entry on page 120); it is caused by inadequate oil and water in the layers of the skin. With radiation especially, the skin may start to peel and/or appear sunburned.

What You Can Do to Help

• Make sure your partner consumes plenty of fluids (two quarts or more) every day.

• Draw a soothing warm bath for your partner sprinkled with mineral or baby oil.

• Encourage your partner to apply mineral oil, baby

oil, or heavier lubricant creams (such as Nivea) immediately after bathing while the skin is still damp in order to retain moisture in the skin. Even better, treat your partner to a massage using an oil or cream for an extrasoothing experience.

• Shop carefully for skin-care products. Moisturizers and mild cleansers do not have to be expensive to be effective: The key moisturizing ingredient in most luxury skin creams is imidazolidinyl urea, which can also be found in less expensive brands in many drug stores.

• Make sure your partner gets regular exercise. Exercise brings blood and other nutrients to the tiny vessels that nourish the skin. Even moderate exercise will bring color and glow back into skin that has become pale and sallow by cancer treatments and too much bed rest.

• Warn your partner against the use of heating lamps, ice packs, hot-water bottles, or any other very hot or very cold liquid, as extreme temperatures will increase skin irritation.

• Suggest that your partner wear only soft cotton clothing that does not bind or rub against the skin. Women should avoid wearing tight-fitting brassieres, girdles, and belts; men should not wear tight, starched collars or close-fitting trousers.

• Ask the physician if hydrocortisone cream would be helpful in reducing your partner's skin inflammation.

• If your partner's skin is very itchy, try applying a paste created from cornstarch and water, which should help reduce the irritation. It is important that your partner not scratch his or her skin, as this may lead to infection.

Warning Signs!

Call your partner's physician if and when

- A skin rash develops (see "Skin Sores," below)
- Skin is itchy, sore, or gets very red and painful to the touch

FALLS

Because some cancer patients become exhausted, confused, weak, and/or dehydrated as a result of their disease and disease treatment, knowing what to do in case of a fall is an important part of being a caregiver. Particularly dangerous situations for someone feeling weak or confused include getting in and out of bed or the bathtub and/or losing one's balance while cooking in the kitchen or while taking a walk alone.

What You Can Do to Help

- Leave your partner where he or she has fallen; moving him or her without knowing the extent of injury can lead to further injury. Do not move your partner if there is fluid draining from his or her mouth, ears, or nose, or if he or she is bleeding. If he or she is unconscious, call 911.
- If your partner is conscious, ask if he or she feels any pain
- Check your partner for cuts, bruises, or areas of swelling

• Apply ice packs to any bleeding area. If the bleeding is caused by a small cut, wash the cut thoroughly with mild soap and water and apply a bandage. If the wound is large, call 911, then attempt to stop the bleeding by applying pressure directly to the injury using a sterilized gauze pad or clean cloth.

• If your partner is uninjured, move him or her to a chair or bed; otherwise call an ambulance immediately.

Warning Signs!

Call your partner's physician—or 911—if and when

• Your partner is unconscious or not breathing
• The cause of your partner's falls have not been determined
• A change in mental status occurs as a result of the fall

FATIGUE

Fatigue can be defined as a chronic state of exhaustion in which a person has less energy to do the things he or she normally does, or wants to do. Those with cancer often find themselves fatigued for any number of reasons. Many people feel very tired during and sometimes after radiation therapy or chemotherapy, perhaps because of the buildup of toxic substances that are released by cancer cells as they die. With radiation therapy healthy cells as well as cancer cells are destroyed, and the body must work hard to repair this damaged tissue. Complications or side effects of the disease treatments, such as anemia and infection, can sap the body of energy as well. Finally, fatigue can be exacerbated by other side effects or symptoms, such as loss of appetite, nausea, vomiting, pain, lack of sleep, and lack of muscle tone due to inactivity. Fortunately fatigue caused by treatment side effects is temporary.

What You Can Do to Help

• You and your partner should have the causes of fatigue diagnosed and treated. If your fatigue is related to anemia, for instance, blood transfusions or iron supplements may be prescribed.

• Help your partner better plan his or her days so that there are plenty of rest periods during which strength and energy can be regained. Many people with cancer want to deny the fact that they are ill by trying to keep to their regular schedules. Forcing themselves to do more than they can manage, however, will only increase their health problems.

• Make sure that your partner gets enough rest and sleep.

Warning Signs!

Call your partner's physician if and when

• Your partner is unable to get out of bed for more than twenty-four hours and was previously able to do so

- There are mental changes accompanying your partner's feelings of lethargy
- The fatigue gets worse or fails to improve after treatment is prescribed by the physician

FEVER

The most common cause of fever is infection caused by bacteria or viruses. In the case of people treated with chemotherapy, fever may sometimes be a reaction of your body to the drug. Your partner may develop a fever several hours after chemotherapy, but his or her temperature should be normal on days when treatment is not administered. It is important that you and your partner keep careful track of when fevers develop, since if they are not related to a chemotherapeutic reaction, they may be a sign of a serious infection.

What You Can Do to Help

- Check your partner's temperature every four hours during the day and evening (do not interrupt sleep unless the fever has been quite high, over 102 degrees F or 39 degrees C).
- Offer your partner plenty of fluids, particularly fruit juices that contain vitamin C (if your partner is able to tolerate them).
- An aspirin substitute containing ibuprophen or acetaminophen will help bring down the fever and help your partner feel more comfortable.

• Give your partner warm sponge baths to reduce the fever and make him or her feel pampered.

Warning Signs!

Contact your partner's physician if and when

• The fever reaches above 101 degrees F (38 degrees C) and does not respond within a few hours to a dose of aspirin substitute

HAIR LOSS

Hair loss may occur because chemotherapy drugs travel throughout the body to kill cancer cells, and some of these drugs damage hair follicles, causing the hair to fall out. Hair can be lost from the eyebrows, eyelashes, and pubic area, as well as the scalp.

Hair loss is very variable. Some people treated for cancer experience it and others do not, even with the same drugs. If hair loss does occur, it usually begins within two weeks of the start of therapy and gets worse one to two months after the start of therapy.

Fortunately hair regrowth often begins even before therapy is completed, usually within three to four months. It should be noted that new growth may be quite different from your partner's pretreatment hair: Curly hair may grow in straight; once-dark-brown hair may grow in lighter; and vice versa.

What You Can Do to Help

• Before treatment begins or at the very start of treatment, encourage your partner to buy a wig or toupee. Do this before hair loss begins so that the wig shop can match your partner's hair color and texture. Obtain a list of wig shops in your area from your partner's doctor or nurse, or from the Yellow Pages. Some health insurance policies cover the cost.

• Proper hair care is extremely important during therapy; the use of gentle shampoos and soft brushes and the avoidance of bleaching, perming, and excessive hair spray can help to minimize the loss of hair, or at least slow the process down.

• You and your partner should talk to the physician about how to minimize hair loss. For some patients, wearing a tight scarf or an ice bag on the head during chemotherapy treatments is possible and will reduce or even eliminate hair loss.

• If your partner does lose hair, don't let him or her get discouraged. Remind him or her that hair will grow back and that today's wigs often cannot be distinguished from natural hair.

INFECTIONS

With chemotherapy healthy white blood cells may be destroyed along with cancerous cells. Without sufficient numbers of white blood cells, your partner is unable to fight infections as efficiently as he or she once was. Having a low white blood cell count (also known as leukopenia) is a common side effect of chemotherapy, and not everyone will develop infections because of it. Your partner's body will replenish the lost cells within four to ten days after chemotherapy is administered; his or her doctor may decide to postpone further chemotherapy until his or her blood cells are replenished. Signs and symptoms of active infection are sore throat, fever, pain, swelling, and eye or ear drainage.

What You Can Do to Help

• Help your partner avoid coming into contact with infectious agents by asking friends and family to postpone visiting if they are ill with colds, coughs, or flus.

• If you know that your partner's blood count is low, you should both avoid going anyplace where large groups of potentially germ-carrying people congregate, such as the movies, church, and shopping malls.

• You should also both wash your hands often to avoid spreading infection.

• Make sure your partner carefully cleans any cut or burn he or she receives.

Warning Signs!

Contact your partner's physician if and when

• Your partner experiences any of the symptoms of an infection
• Your partner runs a fever higher than about 101 degrees F.

LEG CRAMPS

If your partner's cancer or cancer therapy makes it necessary for him or her to remain in bed for long periods of time, he or she may develop leg cramps. Other therapy-related causes of leg cramps include the loss of potassium and calcium that may occur with both chemotherapy and radiation.

What You Can Do to Help

• Encourage your partner to change positions frequently during the day and evening. If he or she is too weak to do so, help him or her shift positions every few hours. This will also help prevent bedsores from developing.

• Make sure that your partner exercises his or her legs in bed by bending and straightening them about ten times twice a day. If your partner is too weak to do so on his or her own, do it yourself, and/or ask a physical therapist for help.

• Apply heat, in the form of a heating pad or hot-water bottle, to the leg in spasm, but cover the leg with a towel first to avoid burning the skin.

• Massage your partner's leg when it is cramping.

• If your partner's leg cramps are due to a mineral imbalance, make sure he or she follows doctor's orders to correct the underlying problem.

Warning Signs!

Contact your partner's physician if and when

- Cramping is not relieved by heat or massage
- Cramping continues for more than six to eight hours, or if the leg becomes swollen or hot to the touch.

MOUTH SORES

Also known as stomatitis, mouth sores are caused by the destruction of the cells of the mouth and throat by chemotherapeutic drugs or by the effects of radiation beams used to treat many head and neck cancers. The mouth, gums, or throat may feel sore, and reddened areas that feel raw may develop. A white or yellow film may coat the mouth, or increased mucus may form. Fortunately mouth sores caused by cancer therapy are temporary and will heal shortly after treatment is completed.

What You Can Do to Help

- Make sure your partner drinks plenty of liquids to keep his or her mouth moist. Warm—not hot—herbal teas are often tolerated best; liquid Jell-O is also often appreciated. Ice chips and sips of cold water can also be soothing.
- Proper dental care is essential. Your partner should use a soft-bristle toothbrush after every meal or snack in

order to remove irritating food particles and to help prevent infections and/or tooth decay.

• If your partner wears dentures, he or she should visit a dentist to make sure they are not irritating the mouth. Dentures may have to be refitted after any surgery to the head or neck.

• Check with your partner's physician to see if there is a medicated mouthwash available by prescription that would be appropriate for your partner's problem. Or mix up your own soothing mouth rinse using a teaspoon of baking soda in one cup of warm water.

• Avoid serving your partner very hot or very cold foods, as they may increase mouth irritation. Bland, cool and soft foods, such as custards, yogurt, lukewarm soups, and eggs, often taste best to someone suffering with mouth sores.

• If solid foods are difficult for your partner to swallow because his or her throat is sore, add gravies, sauces, mayonnaise, or melted butter to soften breads, vegetables, and other hard foods. Ask the physician to prescribe a liquid solution that will numb the throat when swallowed if the problem persists.

• If your partner's room is warmed by dry heat, purchase a humidifier to improve air quality, but be sure to change the water every day to prevent the spread of bacteria.

• Check your partner's mouth for sores twice a day using a small flashlight and a padded tongue blade and report any changes to the physician.

• Encourage your partner to avoid alcohol and tobacco, which will further increase mouth and throat irritation.

Warning Signs!

Contact your partner's physician if and when

- You or your partner first notice sores developing
- Bleeding from the sores occurs
- White patches appear on the tongue or the inside of the mouth.

NAUSEA AND VOMITING

Nausea and vomiting are frequent side effects of chemotherapy and/or radiation therapy on various parts of the body, particularly the digestive-tract organs or the eating center of the brain. Experiencing nausea and vomiting is not an indication of whether or not the chemotherapy or radiation treatments are working to destroy cancer cells.

If chemotherapy or radiation is causing your partner to feel nauseous and/or to vomit, you'll probably find these symptoms occur only within six to twenty-four hours after treatment is administered. Once therapy is discontinued, nausea and vomiting should disappear within a week or two.

It should be noted that just thinking about going for treatment can cause nausea and vomiting in people who have experienced these side effects after previous treatments.

What You Can Do to Help

• Ask your partner's physician to prescribe an antinausea pill or suppository your partner can take before each treatment.

• When your partner is able to eat and keep food down between treatments, be sure to serve him or her foods rich in essential vitamins and minerals that are lost with vomiting, including calcium (cheese, milk, yogurt, and dark, leafy vegetables) and potassium (bananas, tomatoes, oranges, raisins, potatoes, and milk).

• Make sure your partner rests after eating, since activity has a tendency to trigger episodes of nausea.

• Suggest that your partner eat only a small snack before treatment and take only fluids for several hours afterward.

• Avoid serving greasy foods, or foods with high-fiber content because they take too long to leave the stomach.

• Encourage your partner to eat dry crackers or suck on hard candies when nausea occurs in order to prevent dry heaves.

• Keep track of episodes of nausea and vomiting and report them to the physician so that appropriate and effective self-care measures can be taken.

• Offer to cook meals for your partner if food preparation causes him or her to become nauseous (see "Appetite, Loss of," above).

Warning Signs!

Contact your partner's physician if and when

- Vomiting continues for more than twenty-four hours
- Your partner is bloated or has pain before he or she vomits and these symptoms are relieved by vomiting
- Your partner shows any signs of dehydration (sunken eyes, dry skin, dizziness, extreme thirst —see "Dehydration," above)
- You are worried that your partner has aspirated (inhaled) any vomited material
- Blood appears in the vomitus
- Your partner cannot eat any substantial food for more than two days
- Your partner is unable to take his or her medications

PAIN MANAGEMENT

Cancer patients may have pain for a variety of reasons, and it is important to note that not all people with cancer have pain. Pain may be due to the effects of the cancer itself, or it could result from treatment methods.

Pain may be acute or chronic. Acute pain is severe and lasts a relatively short time. It is usually a signal that body tissue is being injured in some way, and the pain generally disappears when the injury heals. Chronic pain, on the other hand, may range from mild to severe and is present to some degree for long periods of time. Cancer pain that lasts a few days or longer may result from

- The tumor causing pressure on organs, nerves, or bone
- Poor blood circulation because the cancer has blocked blood vessels
- Blockage of an organ or tube in the body
- Metastasis, or cancer cells that have spread to other sites in the body
- Infection or inflammation
- Side effects from chemotherapy, radiation therapy, or surgery
- Stiffness from inactivity
- Psychological responses to illness, such as tension, depression, or anxiety

However, whatever the cause, pain *can* be relieved. Several methods are available, including pain medication, nerve blocks, physical therapy, and techniques such as relaxation, distraction, and imagery.

What You Can Do to Help

- Locate and define the pain. Because pain affects each individual in a different way, your partner may have a hard time describing it. The first step is to help your partner identify the pain so that the doctor and you can best treat it. Here are helpful questions to ask:

Where is the pain?

When did it begin?

Is it sharp? Dull? Throbbing? Steady? Intermittent?

Does it prevent you from doing things? What things?

What relieves the pain? What makes it worse?

Is your pain constant? If not, how often does it occur and when?

How long does it last?

How bad is the pain? (In order to help your partner measure the intensity, you may want to use a pain scale that rates the level of pain from 0 to 5, with 0 being no pain and 5 being the worst pain you can imagine.)

• Make sure that your partner's physician is aware of the pain and prescribes appropriate pain medication.

• Create a pain diary. You and your partner should keep careful track of when pain occurs, what may have precipitated its onset, and the behaviors and medications that work best to relieve it. This information will help you and the physician better control pain in the future.

• Distract your partner. Spend time just talking together—about anything other than cancer or pain—rent video movies and watch them with him or her, and/or bring magazines and catalogs your partner can look through without having to concentrate as much as he or she would with a novel or other text.

Warning Signs!

Contact your partner's physician if and when

- Any new, severe pain occurs
- Your partner is unable to consume pain medication by mouth (due to nausea, severe dry mouth or mouth pain)
- The pain is not relieved by prescribed medication
- You or your partner has any questions about how to take the pain medication

SEXUAL PROBLEMS

The treatment of certain cancers, specifically those involving the female and male reproductive and urinary tracts, may directly lead to sexual problems that are quite physical in nature. In Chapter 5, those problems were discussed and some solutions presented.

In addition, however, you and your partner may experience changes in your sexual relationship no matter what type of cancer your partner has. (If you and the person you care for are not married or otherwise sexually involved, pass this information on to your partner and his or her lover.)

With an illness as serious as cancer, both our physical bodies and our emotional makeup undergo a series of changes that often dramatically affect our sexual lives. In addition cancer puts a toll on one's time and energy, often making sex seem like the last thing on a long list of priorities. However, although other aspects of life with cancer may seem more important to you and your partner than sex, intimate behavior is a natural, integral part of all our lives. For your sake, and for your partner's sake, don't ignore it.

As you know, although cancer can attack at any age, the majority of cancer patients are diagnosed after the age of fifty, at a time when both women and men have experienced physical changes that involve their sexual habits. Once a woman enters menopause at about age fifty, for instance, hormonal changes often lessen the production of vaginal lubrication, making sexual relations uncomfortable or painful. Women who undergo hysterectomies and oophorectomies and require hormonal treatment for their cancers are likewise affected by a lack of estrogen. With less estrogen the vaginal wall becomes thinner, and intercourse may feel rough or scratchy.

Older men may find that it takes longer to achieve an erection and that the erection is not as firm as it once was. A decrease in the amount of ejaculate and decreased force of ejaculation may also result from the aging process. This may lead to feelings of inadequacy and a decline in libido. Radiation therapy to the male genital area can cause temporary pain and/or erectile problems.

At any age sexual ability and desire may be affected by a number of physical factors, medication (of any kind) and stress being the most prevalent. In addition to these physical factors, your partner's self-esteem may have taken a blow from the diagnosis of cancer. He or she may feel less attractive and/or "less of a man" or "less of a woman." Your partner may feel afraid of being unable to perform or enjoy sexual relations as much as he or she had before cancer. Your partner may even be afraid that you are staying with him or her out of pity and could never really be sexually attracted to him or her again.

Guilt is perhaps the biggest sexual turnoff of all, and both you and your partner may well have built a wall of guilt between you. Your partner feels guilty, that he or she has become a burden or has become less attractive. You probably feel guilty because you naturally feel resentful of the disease and the time it takes away from your regular life.

Finally, if you are your sexual partner's primary caregiver, you both may have difficulty in discarding your caregiver and patient "roles" for the equality good sexual relations requires. If you must wash your partner's hair for him or her because he or she feels weak after chemotherapy, for example, then seeing your partner as sexually desirable can be quite difficult—and vice versa.

What You Can Do to Help

• Talk to a physician or counselor, preferably with your partner present. There is no one solution to sexual dysfunction, and you and your partner should speak to the physician so that the nature of the problem can be identified and a strategy devised to help you both cope better with your sexual problems.

It may be necessary to press your partner's physician to deal with sexual issues. Unfortunately health care providers often fail to give serious consideration to the sexual issues faced by the chronically ill and their partners. Nevertheless you should make every attempt to gain advice from your partner's primary physician and, if necessary, a referral to a competent sexual therapist.

• Focus first on the physical problems, because they are the ones that are usually easily fixed. Vaginal dryness, which may occur after gynecological surgery or some forms of chemotherapy, can be alleviated by using water-soluble lubricating jellies such as K-Y jelly.

• Try new sexual positions if surgery or treatment has made old positions uncomfortable. If actual penetration is difficult or impossible, look for other alternatives to satisfaction. Mutual masturbation or other means of stimulation are options that should be considered without hesitation if both of you feel comfortable about them. Consider seeking the advice of a therapist if you are unable to break down some of the barriers to communication.

• Be open and honest with your partner and encourage sharing your feelings. Be as direct as you can about your sexual needs and preferences and encourage your partner to do the same.

• Try to plan sexual activity for times your partner is feeling at his or her best. You might think that discussing and planning sexual activity will take the "thrill" of it away. In fact anticipation and planning can add both excitement and self-confidence to your lovemaking. If your partner feels most ill the day after receiving chemotherapy, for instance, it is highly unlikely that he or she will be interested in sex at this time. Choosing a time that works for both you and your partner also allows you to emerge from your roles as caregiver and patient. For that hour or two force yourself to leave your other, caretaking self behind and your partner to cast aside any feelings of illness or disability. Instead become equals in the quest for mutual pleasure.

Most important, both you and your partner should know that you can still touch and embrace without having it necessarily lead to sexual intercourse. In fact sex therapists often impose a "no sex allowed" period, during which their patients refrain from intercourse while they learn other ways of relaxing and feeling intimate with each other. The sexual act is just one part, albeit an important one, of a loving relationship. Enjoy the pleasure that comes from gentle caresses, hugs, and kisses.

• If, after speaking with your partner's and your own physician, you feel you need more help in coping with your sexual problems, seek professional advice from a qualified sex therapist. Try to choose someone who has experience treating cancer patients and their partners; ask your partner's physician for a recommendation.

Warning Signs!

Contact your partner's physician if and when

- Your partner experiences pain with sexual intercourse
- Bleeding occurs
- You and/or your partner have any questions concerning sexual activity or how cancer or cancer treatment may be affecting your relationship

SHORTNESS OF BREATH

Breathing difficulty occurs whenever not enough oxygen is delivered to the body, either because not enough oxygen enters the lungs or because the lungs are unable to deliver oxygen efficiently to the bloodstream. Some drugs used as chemotherapeutic agents may cause damage to lung tissue, making the lungs unable to function properly. Chest pain, rapid pulse, and wheezing may accompany shortness of breath.

If your partner experiences any of these symptoms, it is important that you let the doctor know immediately. If a chemotherapeutic drug is destroying lung tissue, the doctor will replace it with a less toxic medicine. If the damage was not severe, lung tissue can regenerate in time. (If your partner suffers from lung cancer, see Chapter 5 for more information.)

What You Can Do to Help

• If your partner smokes cigarettes, cigars, or pipe tobacco, now is the time for him or her to break the habit. Help in any way you can.

• After receiving advice from the doctor, help your partner make the most out of the lung tissue that is still healthy by taking him or her through regular deep-breathing lessons. Have your partner take three deep breaths through the nose, then hold it while you count to 5. Then ask your partner to cough deeply, using the stomach muscles, as he or she exhales. Repeat the exercise at least once every four hours. These exercises will help keep chest muscles and the diaphragm flexible and strong.

• Make sure your partner conserves as much energy as possible.

• If your partner cannot catch his or her breath and is in a great deal of distress, sit him or her up and tilt the head forward. Instruct your partner slowly and calmly to inhale through the nose and exhale through the lips for twice as long as it took to inhale.

Warning Signs!

Contact your partner's physician if and when

- Your partner first experiences shortness of breath or chest pain
- You hear wheezing or if coughing up of sputum occurs
- Fever occurs

SKIN SORES

If your partner has to remain in bed for any extended period of time, special attention will have to be paid to the condition of his or her skin. When some part of the body lies against a surface such as a mattress for too long, the oxygen flow to that area of the body is stopped and the skin in that area dies, forming painful sores. The tailbone, hips, spine, elbows, heels, and ankles are particularly susceptible to the development of these sores, which can be made worse if rubbed against by sheets or bedclothes.

What You Can Do to Help

• Bathe the sore very carefully with warm water, then cover it with a bandage. Change the bandage at least once a day.
• Make sure your partner changes his or her position in bed several times a day. Use bed pads and soft sheets.
• Take walks or otherwise exercise with your partner as often as possible.
• Keep skin dry to prevent worsening of bed sores.
• Encourage your partner to drink plenty of water and other fluids, which will help keep the skin soft and supple.

Warning Signs!

Contact your partner's physician if and when

• The sore is getting larger
• The sore smells foul
• You notice green or yellow liquid draining from the sore

SLEEP PROBLEMS

Sleep problems can be defined as a change in usual sleeping habits. People who are under treatment for cancer may tire easily and may need to sleep more than usual. Sometimes the opposite problem occurs and insomnia is the problem. Reasons for changes in usual sleeping habits include pain, anxiety, worry, night sweats or other side effects of therapy.

What You Can Do to Help

• It may be necessary for both you and your partner to modify your definitions of "normal" sleep requirements. As we age, we generally require less sleep. If your partner feels refreshed after just four, five, or six hours of sleep, he or she shouldn't try for more—and you shouldn't worry that he or she needs more.

• If your partner wakes up often in the middle of the night, suggest that he or she not try to force himself or herself back to sleep. Instead reading or watching television may help him or her to feel drowsy again.

• Work with your partner to establish a "prebedtime ritual" that will help prepare his or her mind for sleep. A routine of taking a warm bath, having a cup of herbal tea, and/or reading for an hour after getting into bed may make falling asleep easier to do.

• Prepare your partner warm, noncaffeinated drinks such as warm milk with honey before bedtime.

• Encourage your partner to avoid stimulants, such as coffee, tea, cola, or chocolate, especially late in the day.

• Make sure the sleep environment is quiet, attractive, and comfortable.

• Attempt to establish a regular sleeping pattern—naps at the same time every day, bedtime at a regular time every night.

- Give massages or backrubs to relax your partner.
- If your partner has been prescribed medication for pain or sleeplessness by his or her physician, make sure that he or she takes it as directed. Be aware, however, that the use of sleeping pills should be considered only a short-term solution to the problem.

Warning Signs!

Call the doctor if and when

- Your partner's insomnia is accompanied by confusion
- Your partner is unable to sleep despite following the above recommendations

SWALLOWING PROBLEMS

Irritation of the lining of the throat, also known as esophagitis, may be caused by both chemotherapy and radiation therapy and can result in your partner having trouble eating or drinking. Lowered resistance to infection, a common side effect of chemotherapy, often results in treatable infections of the mouth or esophagus, such as thrush. In addition, if your partner has cancer of the mouth, throat, or esophagus, the cancer itself may cause obstruction and irritation; surgery and radiation to treat head and neck cancers also severely affect the ability of the patient to swallow easily and without pain.

What You Can Do to Help

• If your partner's mouth is irritated and sore, make sure you prepare bland foods that are high in calories and protein and soft and smooth in consistency, such as puddings, ice cream, yogurt, and milk shakes.

• Talk to your partner's doctor about adding a high-protein supplement to the diet.

• Mash or blenderize hard foods such as meats and cereal until they form a baby-food-like consistency.

• Your partner may find it more difficult to swallow clear fluids than thicker substances. Try blending fruit with yogurt.

• Experiment with food temperature. Generally foods served at room temperature, rather than very hot or very cold, are most easily tolerated.

• Encourage your partner to avoid alcohol, citrus fruits, crackers, nuts, and spicy foods; all of these substances can cause additional irritation.

• Provide sugar-free hard candies, Popsicles, and sugar-free gum to your partner. Chewing and sucking on these substances may help to stimulate saliva production.

• Make sure your partner keeps regular dentist appointments; in fact he or she may need to see the dentist more often if the mouth is severely affected by cancer and/or cancer therapy.

• Liquid, local pain relievers, such as lidocaine or liquid Tylenol, are available by prescription. Swishing out the mouth with such a solution will ease the tenderness.

• Artificial salivas may relieve feelings of dryness.

Warning Signs!

Call your partner's physician if and when

- Your partner gags or chokes on food more than usual
- Your partner has a severe, persistent sore throat
- Ulcers or sores form on the tongue, cheeks, or palate
- Your partner has difficulty breathing or has chest congestion
- A temperature greater than 100.5 degrees F develops

SWELLING

Also known as edema, swelling involves a buildup of water in body tissues. Both radiation and chemotherapy may cause your partner to retain excess fluid, most notably in the ankles and hands. Your partner may notice that rings are pinching the fingers and/or waistbands on clothing are becoming too tight. If fluid retention becomes severe, the treatment plan may have to be altered to include different chemotherapeutic drugs or lesser amounts of radiation.

What You Can Do to Help

- Keep your partner's feet elevated as much as possible.

- Encourage your partner to wear loose-fitting clothes.
- Restrict the amount of salt in your partner's diet, eliminating as much as possible very salty foods like bacon, nuts, potato chips, and canned meats and vegetables.
- Increase the amount of potassium in the diet by adding apricots, bananas, potatoes, raisins, and unsalted tomato juice.

Warning Signs!

Call your partner's physician if and when

- Your partner is unable to eat for more than a day
- Swelling spreads up the arms or legs
- The belly appears puffy or blown up

WEIGHT GAIN

Although it is much more common for cancer fighters to lose weight during therapy, there are some chemotherapeutic drugs that may increase the fatty tissue in the body. Rounding of the face and fat deposits between the shoulder blades may develop. Some drugs cause the appetite to increase and, coupled with the tendency for the body to retain water (see "Swelling," above), your partner may find himself or herself gaining several pounds during the course of treatment. Fortunately once the treatment is over, the fat deposits disappear and appetite returns to normal within a few weeks.

What You Can Do to Help

• As difficult as it may be, encourage your partner to stay at his or her normal weight by eating low-calorie and low-fat foods.

• As long as your partner is able, he or she should continue to exercise. Even a brisk fifteen-minute walk after dinner will go a long way in helping your partner stay fit. To really help him or her, join in as much as possible.

• Ask a nutritionist (someone recommended by your partner's physician or oncology nurse) to design an eating plan that takes into consideration your partner's individual problems, such as mouth sores, dry mouth, or other side effects that may interfere with the diet.

Warning Signs!

Call your partner's physician if and when

• Your partner gains more than five to ten pounds

WOUNDS AND SCARS

Since surgery remains a first-line treatment for many cancers, you and your partner should learn how to take proper care of the wound and the scar that forms as it heals. In addition to surgery, wounds may be caused by tumor growth inside the body or as a side effect of radiation therapy. The wound may be present only underneath the skin, may affect only the skin surface, or involve both.

What You Can Do to Help

- Make sure you and your partner keep your hands clean whenever you touch the wound or the area around the wound.
- If the wound is bleeding, cleanse well and apply moderate pressure with a cool cloth or ice pack until the bleeding stops. Apply a fresh dressing.
- Clean the wound daily with soap and water, rinse well, pat dry, and apply a fresh dressing as directed by your partner's physician or nurse.
- Do not rub the wound or apply tape directly on the skin around the wound.
- Encourage your partner to eat plenty of citrus fruits (if he or she does not suffer from dry mouth or mouth sores), green leafy vegetables, and protein-rich foods; they all contain vitamins and minerals that promote healing.

Warning Signs!

Call your partner's physician if and when

- The wound bleeds for fifteen minutes or more after you apply pressure
- The wound appears very red or swollen, or if it smells foul
- A greenish-yellow liquid oozes from the wound

- Pain increases or a fever rises to above 100 degrees F

In this chapter general symptoms and side effects of radiation and chemotherapy were discussed, and ways to help alleviate them were offered. In Chapter 7 we concentrate on other tools that can be used in cancer treatment, tools that only your partner has access to—his or her own power of positive thinking.

SEVEN

The Healing Power of Hope

"My mother really surprised me," admits Lois Saunders. "At first she was devastated by the diagnosis of breast cancer. She seemed so overwhelmed when she came to me and asked me to help her through the ordeal. After a long and difficult two years of treatment, I was the one who was overwhelmed—by my mother's strength and dignity."

Isabel, Lois's mother, was sixty-eight years old when she was diagnosed. Her husband had passed away three years previously after a brief but painful struggle with liver cancer. "I think she was terrified that she'd succumb the way my father had. She was so sad before the operation, which was a modified radical mastectomy, that I thought maybe she was going to simply give up."

During surgery Isabel's doctors discovered that breast cancer cells had invaded the axillary lymph nodes, which were removed along with her breast in the procedure. Fearing that errant cancer cells were traveling through her lymph system, her primary physician decided to add chemotherapy to the treatment plan.

"When we found out that the cancer may have

spread, I went into a kind of shock and assumed my mother had too. Instead the news kind of snapped her out of what I thought was a pretty passive mood. Even while she was still in the hospital, I began to see a change in her. It was as if she just decided that she'd be in control of the whole thing. Not that she ordered people around or anything, though she was pretty firm with those of us who tried to make decisions for her or talk about her as if she weren't in the room. It was more like she decided that she 'owned' this cancer; it was hers and she would take care of it in her own way."

As soon as she was able to leave the hospital, Isabel joined a support group for breast cancer patients, women just like her who were coping with the same disease and the same fears. *"My mother had always been a religious woman. She went to church every Sunday and had all of us children baptized. But I never thought of her as spiritual, as feeling that she was part of God. With help from her support group, though, she was able to focus her spiritual energy in a very meaningful way."*

Through her support group Isabel learned some relaxation techniques, techniques that allowed her to recognize the many different emotions she realized she'd been denying, even to herself. Once she identified her fear and anger, she expressed them to the group, releasing them and putting the rest of her life into perspective.

"It wasn't as if everything was suddenly all sunny and positive," Lois remembers. *"But Mother's meditations gave her strength. Every morning she would sit quietly in a chair overlooking the garden and concentrate on getting well. She didn't imagine cancer cells getting*

eaten up by her immune system or anything. She told me she just thought hard about being well and living to see her grandchildren through college."

Last month Isabel's physician found a small tumor in Isabel's other breast, requiring another surgery and a different chemotherapy protocol. "Is my mother discouraged?" asks Lois. "Of course. But through the last few years she's found a kind of inner joy and light that is seeing her through this next battle. I'm grateful that I'll be beside her, learning from her as well as helping her."

"The best inspirer of hope is the best physician." So wrote the nineteenth-century French neurologist Jean Martin Charcot, a doctor as much renowned for his powers of observation as his medical techniques. Today, after several centuries of shunting aside the power of hope in favor of medical technology, more and more modern Western physicians are realizing how important the human spirit is to health and to the battle against disease.

In this chapter we'll discuss some of the groundbreaking research being done in the field of psychoneuroimmunology—the study of how human emotions and the brain may affect the body's ability to fight disease. We'll also look at some of the ways that this potential internal weapon against cancer and other illnesses may be better harnessed by individual patients.

In the past two chapters you've learned some very practical ways that you can physically help your partner deal with the disease that he or she faces. The kind of information presented in this chapter, however, is far less practical. Hope and spiritual peace are not things that can be imparted from one person to another, but rather spring from within an individual's own mind and heart.

As stated many times throughout this book, however, one of your primary duties as a caregiver is to gather information and present options. By better understanding the possible impact your partner's emotions may have on the course of his or her cancer therapy—and sharing this knowledge with your partner—you will be able to create an environment in which hope and positive energy have the chance to flourish.

RESURRECTING THE MIND-BODY CONNECTION

A wife falls ill and passes away within just a few months of her husband's death. A businessman working overtime under the stress of an impending deadline develops a head cold he cannot shake. A grandmother, like Isabel, seems to will herself to live long enough to see her granddaughter receive a college degree. An otherwise happy and satisfied young man succumbs to clinical depression as he struggles to control a nagging case of chronic asthma.

Chances are you've been witness to one or more examples like those described above in which the state of someone's mind appears to directly affect his or her health. In some ways such a connection seems obvious and commonsensical. But because of the way that Western medical science has developed during the past four or five hundred years, the link between mind and body has been effectively severed, at least within the realm of conventional medicine.

However, evidence that there is indeed a powerful mind-body connection has steadily mounted. One of the oldest scientific proofs of the interdependence of mind and body is the well-known "fight-or-flight response." When we feel fear, our bodies react in very physical ways, ways that can be measured. Our blood pressure rises, our heart rate soars, our palms sweat. Blood rushes to our muscles, providing them with the extra oxygen they'll need to mount a physical fight or to run away. We may not be able to isolate and identify "fear" within our bodies, but we can measure what fear causes our bodies to do.

Slowly but surely doctors throughout the Western world have begun to accept the notion that emotions can influence—if not cause or cure—the disease process. In the 1970s a technique called biofeedback emerged that helped further prove the connection. This method developed after studies showed that animals could control their autonomic functions, including blood pressure and heart rate, by being given a reward or a punishment. Physicians adapted those findings to design ways for humans to control unconscious functions through conscious thought.

That the mind and body are linked is also evident in what is called the placebo effect. Simply put, the placebo effect postulates that if we believe strongly enough that a cure will work, we are more likely to be cured—even if the treatment has no basis in scientific fact. An individual who expects to get well by following her physician's advice and taking a pill, for instance, is quite apt to get well even if the pill she takes is made of sugar. By the same token, if that woman has no belief that the cure prescribed will make her well, it is likely that she will fare poorly, even if the substance is potent.

This is hardly to say that all quack cures for cancer—such as laetrile, for instance—will work if we only believe in them strongly enough. Indeed, thousands of people have died, some of them needlessly, by believing in such false miracles. Nevertheless there does appear to be a strong link between what our minds believe and how our bodies behave. Until recently, however, the clear if largely immeasurable connection between the mind and body has largely been ignored by organized Western medicine.

Today, though, a new science is emerging, one that intends to show that the interdependent nature of the mind and body is the key to understanding both health and disease.

THE SCIENCE OF PSYCHONEUROIMMUNOLOGY

One of the most promising avenues of mind-body research brings together three specialties that once worked in almost complete isolation from one another —psychology (the study of behavior and the mind), neurology (the study of the nervous system), and immunology (the study of the immune system, the disease-fighting cells of the body).

Recent experiments performed under the auspices of

this new science have shown startling, unexpected results. One study conducted at the University of California at Los Angeles, for instance, involved actors, individuals who by nature and training are able to elicit from themselves strong emotions on cue. As the actors experienced a certain emotion, researchers tested their hormones and blood to see what if any changes occurred. They were surprised to find an increase in activity of certain white blood cells—the cells that make up the immune system. This increase in activity occurred no matter what kind of emotion—positive or negative —was evoked.

It would seem, at first glance, that having an emotional crisis could actually work to fight disease since it triggers the immune system to take action. But researchers postulate that the immune system could become overworked if constantly stimulated, eventually losing its effectiveness and leaving the body open to disease. This would explain why illness tends to occur when we are under prolonged stress.

Exactly how thoughts and emotions act on immune-system cells is still not fully understood. One avenue of research involves nerve cells called neurotransmitters and immune-system cells. Long considered completely unconnected, it now appears that the immune system and nervous system communicate regularly by means of neurotransmitters, nerve cells that carry messages from the brain. Although still under investigation, these findings may show that the brain (the core of the central nervous system) is capable of triggering the immune system to perform in certain ways—the same way that the brain, when it senses fear, can tell the heart to beat faster.

Another connection between the brain and the immune system is composed of chemicals called neuropeptides. Like neurotransmitters, these chemicals were once thought to exist only in the brain but have since been found throughout the body. According to current theory, these information chemicals may be the physical representations of emotions and feelings. Neuropeptides control, for instance, the opening and closing of blood vessels in the face. When you suddenly feel embarrassed, these chemicals are responsible for the blush that rushes to your cheeks.

What all of these studies show is that, at least in theory, the distinction made between body and mind is a false one. Instead the mind exists throughout our body as well as in our brain and, in the best possible world, treatment for disease should take that fact into consideration.

On a practical level several studies have shown not only that the mind-body connection exists but that it may be a very powerful force in fighting disease. In 1989 the results of a study confirmed what many physicians and patients had believed for some time—that the emotional support provided by cancer support groups affected in a positive way the outcome of treatment. Dr. David Spiegel, a psychiatrist at Stanford University, divided a group of eighty-six women, all of whom had metastatic breast cancer. One group was given standard medical care—surgery, chemotherapy, and radiation. The members of the other group received the same therapy but were also asked to meet once a week in a group-therapy session in which emotions—often dismissed by physicians concentrating on the strictly physical aspects of cancer—were expressed, discussed, and confronted.

The immediate effects surprised few people: The women who had the support of fellow cancer patients and a qualified leader reported fewer symptoms of depression, anxiety, and pain than those in the other group. After all, they had more opportunities to express their emotions and find solutions to problems.

What did surprise Dr. Spiegel and other physicians were the long-range effects of support groups. Several years later Spiegel made a startling discovery: Those who took part in the group psychotherapy had lived twice as long after they entered the study as the group that received only standard medical care.

Another study, conducted in the 1980s at the Malignant Melanoma Clinic in San Francisco by psychologist Lydia Temoshob, showed similar results. Cancer patients who displayed an overreaching need to be in control and who were unable to express their emotions (whom Temoshob termed Type C patients) did not respond as well to treatment as did their more expressive and more relaxed counterparts.

One of the most famous and well-documented studies of the mind-body connection and cancer patients was performed in the late 1970s by Dr. O. Carl Simonton and his wife, Stephanie Matthews-Simonton. The Simontons developed a meditation and visualization program to help people with cancer tap into the power of their own emotions. In an interview for the book *The Practical Encyclopedia of Natural Healing,* Dr. Simonton stated his beliefs this way: "You [the cancer patient] may actually, through a power within you, be able to decide whether you will live or die, and if you choose to live, you can be instrumental in choosing the *quality* of life you want." In 1979 the Simontons published a study that showed that cancer patients who were helped to use their minds and emotions to alter the course of their cancer lived *two times* longer than those who received medical treatment alone.

Although these and other studies show encouraging results, we are still not sure how to use this information to treat or prevent diseases such as cancer; but scientists across the country and around the world continue to search for answers.

TECHNIQUES FOR FOSTERING THE MIND-BODY CONNECTION

Whether or not thoughts and emotions will ever be able to fight disease is still unknown, and certainly no reputable physician would tell you or your partner that cancer can be cured simply by positive thinking. But it has been shown that patients who are relaxed, optimistic, feel supported by family and other cancer patients, and are aware of their own inner emotional or spiritual life tend to feel better and fare better than those who feel helpless and out of control.

Several techniques have been developed that may help your partner better participate in his or her own recovery.

Relaxation

Learning to relax and relieve tension is important to the person with cancer for many reasons. Needless to say, feeling relaxed simply feels better than feeling tense. In addition, as discussed above, constant stress and anxiety may cause the immune system to become overstimulated and thus less able to fight disease. Furthermore relaxing may also help aid in another important mind-body technique—visualization—which is described below.

Finally, mastering any task tends to make us feel proud and more confident. If your partner can learn to truly relax, even during such a stressful time, he or she may gain a sense of control over his or her body that he or she may have felt was lost forever because of the cancer.

There are many relaxation exercises that will help relieve tension and put your partner into a relaxed state. Offer the following suggestions to him or her:

• *The inhale/tense, exhale/relax method.* First, lie or sit in a comfortable position and close your eyes. Take a deep breath and, while doing so, tense all of the muscles in the body, from your feet to your eyelids. Hold the position for five seconds. Then, as you slowly exhale, release your muscles all at once and feel your body go limp. Breathe normally and feel how relaxed your body is in this position.

• *The breathing-meditation method.* Again, lie or sit in a comfortable position and close your eyes. In this exercise the purpose is to concentrate only on the sound and feeling of your own breathing and thus induce a kind of hypnotic state. First choose a pair of words, such as "in" and "out" or "one" and "two," or "peace" and "strength." As you inhale, think to yourself, *One;* as you exhale, think, *Two.* Repeat this over and over, breathing in about seven times a minute. Think only of those words and the sound of your breath as you breathe in and out. After ten minutes or so you should feel relaxed and refreshed.

Visualization

Once your partner is able to put himself or herself into a relaxed, calm state at will, he or she may want to try what is known as visualization or imagery. This technique will use your partner's imagination to create soothing mental images—such as a sun-filled stretch of beach surrounded by warm, blue water—that will deepen the state of relaxation. Another way of using imagery and visualization is to depict a certain process or goal, such as chemotherapeutic drugs entering the bloodstream and destroying cancer cells.

Or, like Isabel in the case study that opened this chapter, your partner may want to picture a special event in the near or distant future that he or she fears illness will prevent him or her from attending. In the visualization your partner can place himself or herself at the event, smiling and laughing. Concentrating on that image may help him or her get through therapy with more energy and good health.

No matter what image is evoked, your partner will be attempting to use his or her mind to direct the body to do something positive to fight the cancer. (The Simontons, mentioned earlier in this chapter, published a book called *Getting Well Again*, in which more specific meditation and visualization techniques are described. Please see "Appendix 1: Resources" for more information.) Again, the feeling of control and participation that comes with this exercise is every bit as important as the actual physical results.

Faith

It is important for your partner to *believe* that the battle against cancer can be fought and won. Whether God is the one to carry the sword, or your partner's own internal spirit, or the techniques of modern medicine, or some combination of all three, your partner must try to have faith that he or she can be well again or at least live out what is left of life with dignity and satisfaction.

What You Can Do to Help

The information in this chapter was written to help you better understand the connection between your partner's emotions and his or her fight against cancer. As stated earlier, there is little you can do about your partner's inner belief system; you cannot force your partner to believe in a higher power or to practice visualization or relaxation techniques if it is not in his or her nature to do so.

There are, however, some steps you can take to provide your partner with a peaceful, hopeful, and supportive environment.

Restore Control

One of the most distressing, and stress-producing, aspects of cancer and cancer therapy is the loss of control cancer patients often feel, especially during the initial treatment phase. Not only do they often suffer side effects that make them unable to perform their usual tasks, they also feel helpless, unable to affect the course of the disease in any way.

The more control over his or her life your partner can exert, the more confident and able to fight he or she will feel. Resist the temptation to take over simple daily chores, such as washing the dishes or doing the laundry, if your partner is able to do them as before. Encourage your partner to become a partner in his or her health care team, and make sure that he or she is included in important household decision-making whenever possible.

Hope with Your Partner

No matter what your partner's prognosis is, neither one of you should ever give up hope or lose heart. Even if your partner's cancer is terminal, hope and positive energy will help make the coming months easier to bear and more fulfilling for both of you. If the prognosis is good, encourage your partner to make plans for the future. Help him or her come up with a list of both short-term goals and long-term dreams and plans and ways you both can work to meet them.

Provide a Peaceful Environment

Coping with cancer and cancer treatment is often painful, time-consuming, and energy-sapping. Although isolating your partner from ordinary daily chaos will eventually do more damage than good, it is possible for you to create a special time and space for your partner —a place to which he or she can retreat for peace and quiet for at least part of every day. If possible, transform a former sewing room or study into a permanent meditation area for your partner. If space is a problem, designate certain times in every day in which the kitchen, living room, or bedroom is reserved for your partner alone.

In addition to a physical place, your partner needs another kind of space in his or daily environment—the emotional space to grow and change and react to the sometimes awful, sometimes joyful new feelings that come from fighting cancer.

Find Support for Your Partner

As discussed above, the Spiegel study conducted during the 1980s proved that emotional support provided by group therapy has a beneficial effect on cancer treatment and survival rates. What accounts for the powerful effect that a supportive environment has on physical health remains a mystery. Perhaps the isolation and desolation felt by many cancer patients who choose to go it alone could well undermine the status of the immune system over the long term. Or the reverse could be true: The release of emotions in a supportive environment may trigger positive immune-system activity that we are as yet still unable to measure.

Needless to say, it is important that your partner be aware that support groups are an integral part of the fight against cancer. Encourage your partner to contact and visit a support group near his or her home or hospital (see "Appendix 1: Resources").

With the possible exception of parts of Chapter 1, the centerpiece of every discussion in this book has been the health and welfare of your partner. In Chapter 8 you'll discover that your health and welfare are important, too, and learn ways you can protect yourself from becoming ill, exhausted, or just plain frustrated.

EIGHT

Taking Care of Yourself

"My daughter and her ten-year-old son moved in with me about six months ago," sixty-five-year-old James Morgan recounts, *"right after Melissa had surgery for invasive cervical cancer. She was divorced and I couldn't see her doing this by herself. I felt so bad for her; she was in so much pain and so scared."*

Melissa Klein was diagnosed with cervical cancer when she was just thirty-eight years old. Since she'd given birth to her son, Jason, she'd neglected her own yearly checkups and hadn't seen a gynecologist for a Pap smear for more than five years. By the time the cancer was discovered, it had invaded much of her pelvic cavity. A complete hysterectomy was recommended, along with chemotherapy and radiation treatments.

"She resisted moving in with me, and who can blame her?" admits James. *"She'd been on her own for twenty years, and her mother died a few years ago. But Melissa's a smart girl and she knew she had quite a fight on her hands, so she sublet her apartment, stored her things, and moved herself and Jason in.*

"At first I was grateful I could be of help. I'm retired

and have lots of time on my hands. I drove Jason across town twice a day so that he could go to his old school, visited Melissa every day at the hospital, then helped her recover at home. I even put up with her bad moods and Jason's television habit without feeling too much discomfort myself."

But as the weeks turned into months, James began to realize he was losing more and more of himself to his caregiving duties. *"It felt awful to complain, even to myself, that I no longer had time to spend a whole day at the golf course or to stay out late with my buddies at a poker game. After all, my daughter was sick and she and my grandson needed me. But I was getting frustrated."*

Fortunately one of James's good friends had spent time as a caregiver himself and gave James some valuable advice. *"Steve told me to get myself to a support group to find out how other caregivers got through this with their sanity intact. And Steve should know. His wife had Parkinson's disease for more than fifteen years, and he told me he spent every minute of the day and night with her, especially as the disease got worse. He never took any care of himself, and it wasn't until he was diagnosed with walking pneumonia that he realized how much it was taking out of him. He finally went to a support group for PD caregivers and found out how normal his problems were and how much help there was for him. So I did the same thing."*

Through James's support group he learned about the visiting nurses' program that would send someone to the home to care for his daughter several hours a week. He also found out that the worst of the treatment was *probably over. "Someone with a sister with cervical cancer diagnosed in the same stage that Melissa's was told me that—as long as the cancer didn't recur—she should start getting better and better from now on. Whether that's really true or not, it made me feel great to have somebody to share with."*

James has now learned to take a little time for himself every day. Jason now takes a bus one way, and as Melissa gets a little stronger, she's beginning to take on more chores around the house. James still feels better staying pretty close to home, but he's no longer in danger of losing his health or happiness to his caregiving responsibilities.

The task you have undertaken—that of providing loving and sensitive care to someone suffering from cancer—is not an easy one. As James has discovered, the responsibilities often feel overwhelming, and your own life can seem to be slipping away from you. It is important that you gain an understanding of your own needs and how to balance them with those of your partner; needless to say, you'll be of no use to anyone if your own emotional or physical health becomes impaired during the course of your caregiving duties.

As we discussed in Chapter 1, few people who become caregivers are free to devote their entire selves to their new duties. Most people juggle many roles at the same time; even James, who was retired, had responsibilities as a grandfather and friend in addition to those related to caregiving.

Women are at special risk when it comes to caregiving: Although an equal number of men and women suffer from cancer, a disproportionate number—more than two thirds—of caregivers are women. There are many reasons for this sex-based discrepancy, including the fact that caregiving has traditionally been a woman's role. There is the added factor of age: Men tend to die at a younger age than women, leaving their wives alone. When a widow falls ill with cancer or another disease, responsibility for her care is likely to fall to her daughter or daughter-in-law.

Indeed today's woman, no matter her age, has learned to become a consummate juggler. She is wife, mother, homemaker, employee, employer, daughter, and ultimately primary caregiver. Not only may she care for the ill in her immediate family, but she may feel an obligation to care for her parents, parents-in-law, and secondary relatives as well. It is not uncommon for a young woman, divorced, working full-time, and raising her children alone, to take on the responsibility of caring for her mother or father as well.

Of course, as James Morgan's story illustrates, men are not immune either. Whether you are a man, woman, child, or sibling, you've accepted a burden that may be placing your own health at risk.

EVALUATING YOUR EMOTIONAL STATE

To help you gain some perspective on your role as a caregiver, take a moment to finish the following statements:

- The most *stressful* thing about caring for someone with cancer is _____.
- The most *irritating* thing about caring for someone with cancer is _____.
- The most *exhausting* thing about caring for
  someone with cancer is _____.
- The most *rewarding* thing about caring for
  someone with cancer is _____.
- The most *frightening* thing about caring for
  someone with cancer is _____.

If you've completed these statements honestly, it is likely that you've learned something new about caregiving. Perhaps the negative aspects are really not so upsetting when you look at them clearly, or perhaps you were unable to think of anything positive to say at all. If your answers trouble or confuse you in any way, you should consider attending a support group and sharing your concerns with other members. Or, at the very least, you should discuss your thoughts with your partner and/or his or her primary physician.

Now answer these questions yes or no:

- Do you get five to six hours of uninterrupted
  sleep most nights? _____
- Can you arrange to be alone for some portion of
  every day? _____
- Is there someone you could/would call for help
  at two A.M.? _____
- Is there one friend or family member who could/
  would loan you money if you were in financial
  trouble? _____

- Is there anyone in your life who fully understands the day-to-day trials you experience?_____

If you answer no to more than one or two questions, you may be heading toward caregiver burnout—a form of emotional and physical exhaustion associated with a total commitment to and immersion in a job or cause. To avoid burnout, you've simply got to remember to *take care of yourself first.*

THE SIX SECRETS TO CAREGIVER SANITY

Secret 1. Take Time for Yourself

As mentioned several times throughout this book, it's easy to lose yourself to your partner and other people who depend on you. As pressing as your caregiving and other responsibilities may be, it is important that you carve out a few hours every day to concentrate on your own needs and pleasures:

- At least once a week treat yourself to a special lunch out, a softball game with your friends, a manicure, a movie, a soothing bubble bath.
- Make sure you maintain your own interests or develop new ones that have nothing whatsoever to do with your partner or with cancer. Although now is probably not the time to embark on a difficult or time-consuming new venture, there are plenty of interesting opportunities that will keep you relatively close to

home. Take an adult-education class once a week in a subject that interests you; resume an old hobby, such as knitting or stamp collecting; perhaps bring a new pet into the home that you, your family, and your partner can enjoy.

• Volunteer your expertise and commitment. Many caregivers find it particularly rewarding to donate a few hours a week to a worthy cause, especially during the times when cancer therapy is routine or their partners are in remission. Some choose to counsel other caregivers of cancer patients, while others devote themselves to another cause that holds special meaning for them.

Secret 2. Eat Well

More than twenty-five hundred years ago the Greek physician and philosopher Hippocrates declared, "Thy food be thy remedy." Today, as we approach the twenty-first century, those words ring with particular urgency and truth. Every day the connection between what we eat and the state of our health becomes clearer and more well defined.

Food is the fuel your body uses to perform its functions. Every day some of your cells die and others are created to replace them. Every day millions of major and minor miracles—the beating of your heart, the digestion of food, the processing of information in the brain—take place within the chemistry lab that is your body. And the catalysts for these processes are the nutrients in the food you eat every day.

Choosing the right foods to eat as well as the right amounts is a highly individual matter. Depending on many different factors, your body requires special ingredients to perform its many functions. A woman who is pregnant, for instance, requires more calories than a woman who has passed through menopause. An athlete's diet may consist of more protein, carbohydrates, and calories than a man with a sedentary job.

Creating an eating plan that takes your special needs into consideration goes far beyond the scope of this book. But there are a few rules you can follow that will help you get the right amount of nutrition—without taking in too many calories—even during this difficult period:

• Take a look at the Food Guide Pyramid issued by the U.S. Department of Agriculture. It provides information about how much and what kinds of foods you should eat every day. If you have questions about the Pyramid or about proper nutrition for yourself or your partner, talk to your partner's physician and dietary counselor.

• Concentrate on eating at least five servings of fruits and vegetables every day.

• Choose whole-grain breads and cereals.

• Limit the amount of fat you consume to less than 30 percent of your daily caloric intake.

• If you find you are gaining weight, as many homebound, stressed-out caregivers do, keep a food diary for a few days or a week. In it note not only what foods you are eating and when but *why* you eat. Do you eat more when your partner is in the hospital? Is food a comfort to you when you are worried or sad? Just keeping track of the emotions behind your eating may help you learn to have better control.

• Avoid eating fast foods on the run. It's often easiest to grab a cheeseburger on the way to visit your partner in the hospital or on your way to or from the pharmacy rather than prepare a balanced meal at home—especially if your partner cannot tolerate cooking odors or has a restricted diet. But fast food is not the answer unless you choose carefully. Opt for plain burgers without cheese or special sauces, always order a salad (preferably with low-calorie dressing), and pick up an apple or orange rather than an apple pie or orange soda.

Secret 3. Exercise Regularly

The importance of regular exercise to your general health cannot be overestimated. In fact in the fall of 1992 the American Heart Association formally designated inactivity as one of the four top risk factors for the development of heart disease and stroke, America's number-one killers. Nevertheless only about 40 percent of all Americans exercise on a regular, sustained basis.

If you embark upon a sensible exercise plan, you can significantly lower your risk of stroke, hypertension, heart disease, and myriad other diseases that are influenced by obesity—a familiar result of inactivity—such as breast cancer, colon cancer, and diabetes. In addition vigorous exercise is likely to make you feel better emotionally: Your brain is fed by thousands of tiny capillaries; the more blood coursing through them to feed the brain, the more mentally alert and emotionally satisfied you may feel.

If you're just beginning to embark on your caregiving duties, now is probably not the time to begin a complicated or time-consuming exercise plan unless you've been an avid exerciser in the past. Here are a few tips to help get you started on something simple and basic:

• Check with your own physician before starting any new exercise program, especially if you haven't been active in the recent past.

• Concentrate on getting aerobic exercise, which will improve cardiovascular health by forcing the body to deliver ever-larger amounts of oxygen to working muscles. (Anaerobic exercise attempts to strengthen individual muscles.) Walking, jogging, aerobic dance or step classes, and bicycling are just some of your options.

• Always spend a few minutes gently—very gently—stretching your muscles and running in place to warm them up before you begin the main portion of your exercise routine.

• Try to reach your target heart rate and exercise at that level for about twenty minutes a session, three times a week. Your target heart rate is the rate at which your heart must work to provide benefits to the cardiovascular system. (Your target heart rate is between 60 and 80 percent of your maximum heart rate; maximum heart rate is calculated by subtracting your age from 220. The average fifty-year-old would have a maximum heart rate of 220 minus 50, or 170; the target heart rate would then be from 102 to 136 beats per minute.) Work up to this goal slowly, over a period of several weeks.

• If aerobic workouts are not your cup of tea, there is good news. New research indicates that exercise doesn't have to be cardiovascular or even continuous to have important health benefits. You can make gardening, social dancing, or housework part of your exercise regimen. The key is to exercise moderately thirty minutes a day, five to six days a week. Short bursts of ten or fifteen minutes do count toward your daily half-hour quota.

• Choose an activity you enjoy. The time you spend exercising should not seem like another chore in your already overbooked day. Instead it should help you relieve physical and emotional tension and provide you with pleasure. Try several different activities until you find one that's right for you.

• Seek convenience. Time is at a premium in your life right now, so joining a health club across town is probably a self-defeating plan. Find a place or an activity that fits into your life easily; perhaps running around the high school track or using an exercise videotape at home would be easier for you than attempting to join a class that meets at a set time.

Secret 4. Get Enough Sleep

If you have difficulty sleeping, review your daily and bedtime routines carefully, then reread the tips offered in the "A-to-Z Guide" for hints on getting a better night's sleep (see page 149).

Secret 5. Avoid Depression

A special danger to caregiving partners is falling into a depression that threatens their health and self-esteem.

Obviously, taking care of someone with cancer, someone you love who may not survive, is likely to provoke despair and grief. Indeed, experiencing moments or even days when you feel completely overwhelmed by sadness and helplessness is quite normal and in many ways exhibits a healthy response to the challenges faced by a caregiver. However, when these feelings persist and cause radical changes in your day-to-day life, you may require medical intervention to help you cope.

Without a doubt your best protection from the blues is to stay active and involved in activities *other than caregiving*. Find a new hobby or join a health club. Learn to cook Chinese food or take a writing class. As trivial as these activities may seem when you're feeling low, simply getting out and breathing fresh air—both physically and intellectually—is the very best prescription for you to follow.

If your feelings of sadness, loss, and low self-esteem persist, it's essential that you treat your symptoms seriously. If you haven't been able to get yourself up and out of the doldrums, take the time to answer these questions. Have you been experiencing any of the following symptoms for more than a day or two at a time?

_____ Insomnia or excessive sleepiness
_____ Loss of appetite and weight loss
_____ Low energy level
_____ Loss of self-esteem
_____ Decreased productivity
_____ Decreased attention span or increased confusion
_____ Withdrawal from social interaction

_____ Loss of enjoyment, even in activities that
once brought you pleasure

_____ Frequent bouts of irritability or anger

_____ Self-reproach or inappropriate guilt

_____ Recurrent thought of suicide and death

_____ Sense of helplessness and gloom

If you have answered in the affirmative to three or
more of these questions, you may be suffering from depression. If so, you should seek help from your physician immediately. Unlike normal feelings of sadness and
grief, depression is a serious condition frequently requiring medical intervention. If you suffer from true depression, your doctor will most likely prescribe an an-
tidepressant, such as Elavil or Prozac, that is designed to
influence brain chemistry in order to lighten your dark
moods. These drugs should be taken only under the
continued care of a physician or psychiatrist.

Secret 6. Find and Accept Support and Practical Help

Nothing can match the healing power of empathy
and compassion, two qualities found in abundance at
your local American Cancer Society– or hospital-spon-
sored support group. In Chapter 7 you learned the direct effect support groups appear to have on cancer patients' ability to fight their disease; although similar
research has not been done with caregivers, we can assume that comfort and support are equally protective of
their health as well.

If your partner is severely disabled by his or her cancer, you may need to find more sustained and regular

help at some point—and that point should be *before* you become physically ill or emotionally overwrought. As soon as you notice that you no longer have time for yourself or are feeling constantly exhausted, take some of the burden off your shoulders. There are a number of options available to you. Take advantage of one or more of the following:

• *Family and friends.* Resist the impulse to tell the people in your life that you "can handle everything." If you do this often enough, many of them may take you at your word: No longer does your daughter offer to take her father to the hospital for his radiotherapy appointments, nor does your neighbor suggest that she do your grocery shopping when she does her own, thereby giving you time to take a nap. Nevertheless chances are that they would still be happy to help you out—if you'd only ask. As difficult as it may be for you, pick up the phone and call, keeping in mind that your health and the health of your partner are in jeopardy if you don't.

• *Home care.* If your partner is severely disabled, you can hire health care professionals—physical therapists and nurses, among others—to come to your home on an hourly, daily, or weekly basis. This allows your partner to get the needed care as well as giving you a little time on your own. Depending on your insurance or form of government assistance, some or all of this home care may be covered.

• *Hospice care.* If your partner has been diagnosed with a terminal cancer, you may decide that this approach—which provides care and comfort at home or

in an institution during the last several months of life—
is best for both of you. In Chapter 9 you'll read more
about hospice care and how to become involved with
such a program.

NINE

Coping with Death and Dying

"My wife is the one that encouraged the whole idea,"
Peter Fitzgerald recalls. "My father was seventy, diag-
nosed with advanced prostate cancer that had already
spread to the bone and liver, and he had only about
eight months to live. I was devastated, but Rebecca
really helped me pull myself together and make some
decisions."

Peter's father, Oscar, lived about an hour and a half
away, just across the state border, in an apartment he
rented after his own wife passed away a few years be-
fore. "We were never really close as I was growing up,"
Peter recalls, "but since Mom died, we'd been seeing a
lot of each other. I think I got to know him pretty well,
and I knew he didn't want to die alone in a hospital
somewhere."

Following the diagnosis Peter and his father talked a
lot about what was about to happen. "I felt cheated and
angry that just when we were finally getting close, I was
going to lose him. It took me a while to get past that
anger. As for Dad, he went about making plans for his
funeral and making jokes about how much fun he

wanted us to have at the wake, but I don't think he really accepted it until the doctor stopped the radiation treatments, saying that there really wasn't any point since the cancer had spread so fast and so far."

Peter knew that plans for his father's last few months of life needed to be made. *"I talked to the social worker at the hospital where he was diagnosed and found out about hospice care. We were very lucky; there was a terrific program run by our local hospital that accepted my dad and gave my whole family lots of practical help and, frankly, emotional support when we needed it.*

"But it was tough. My father was in a lot of pain and needed constant care, especially as the illness wore on. My children, who are ages six and eleven, were a little frightened and sad that their grandfather was so sick, but they also got a little frustrated and angry that their lives were turned upside down. And my wife—well, she took the brunt of it. She wasn't working at the time, and it fell to her to do most of the day-to-day dirty work. I'll never be able to thank her enough for making my father's last days so peaceful."

At the end the Fitzgeralds decided that Oscar would be best served in the hospice ward of the hospital. *"We agonized about moving him, but it seemed best for everyone. The ward was decorated in a homey way, no sterile, hospital white. And the visiting hours were basically whatever we wanted them to be. During the last week of his life I slept in a bed next to his, and both my wife and I were there with him, holding his hands while he died. I wouldn't trade that moment—or the five months he spent living with us—for the world."*

During the past several decades medical science has made great strides in the treatment of cancer. As cited in Chapter 1, well over 50 percent of all newly diagnosed cancers are successfully cured today. The downside of that story, however, is that treatment for cancer ultimately fails nearly 50 percent of the time. More than 500,000 people die every year from one type of cancer or another; one out of every three Americans will eventually die of cancer.

These statistics are not meant to frighten you: If your partner's prognosis is positive, you both should fight it with every ounce of energy and commitment you can muster and believe that you can beat the disease. On the other hand if your partner's prognosis is poor, it is important to know that neither of you are alone, that there are thousands of other cancer fighters and their caregivers who are facing the same devastating reality. More important, there are coping strategies, and counselors who can help make them work for you, that can help ease the pain and grief you both will feel in the coming months.

COMING TO TERMS WITH IMPENDING DEATH

In Chapter 1 you read about the coping stages that come with a diagnosis of a serious illness such as cancer. By now it is likely that you and your partner have passed through many if not all of them on your way to a positive recovery.

There may come a time, however, when you must face the fact that treatment has failed and that your partner will succumb to this disease. Or perhaps you're reading this already knowing that your partner's cancer is terminal. In either case it is important that you familiarize yourself with the coping stages connected specifically with death and dying so that you can help guide your partner through this difficult time.

Dr. Elisabeth Kübler-Ross, a Swiss-born doctor and one of the pioneers in the study of death, defined the stages of grief in a groundbreaking book, *On Death and Dying,* published in the 1970s. Her work remains the standard reference for anyone trying to cope with a terminal illness. According to Kübler-Ross, a dying person generally passes through five stages before death: denial, anger, bargaining, depression, and acceptance. Keep in mind that not everyone experiences every stage, nor in the order given.

Also keep in mind that although this chapter focuses on the ways that you can help your partner cope with a terminal diagnosis, you'll be deeply affected too. Make sure that your emotional needs are met by talking with a counselor or your own family physician or clergyman.

You may notice that some of the stages involved in coping with death and dying are quite similar to the ones described in Chapter 1 dealing with the diagnosis. In this case, however, these stages are likely to be perceived and dealt with in very different ways by both you and your partner.

Denial

Even if your partner has traveled a long road of failed treatments before receiving a terminal prognosis, he or she may attempt—with every ounce of his or her being —to deny that death is approaching. And if the cancer was diagnosed at a very advanced stage, when any treatment would prove futile, the prognosis may be even more difficult for your partner to accept.

Denial takes many forms. Some people refuse to believe the results of the medical tests and thus deny themselves the chance to take medicine or receive treatment that may help them feel better and perhaps live longer. Others, such as Oscar in the case study, appear to accept that they are dying by cooperating with doctors and even making arrangements for their funerals, but deny the true reality to themselves.

As discussed in Chapter 1, denial can be a very positive stage, allowing your partner to filter in the reality little by little. A brief period of denial may be helpful to you as well, since it may keep you from being overwhelmed by emotion while there are still organizational and caregiving chores to be done.

What You Can Do to Help

As long as denial does not interfere with your partner's medical therapy or ability to make important decisions, you should not force the issue. Instead make yourself available as a sounding board; listen patiently to your partner as he or she begins what may be a long journey to acceptance.

Anger

Needless to say, a quite natural reaction to a poor prognosis is pure, unadulterated anger. After all, your

partner has been told that his or her life will be short-
ened, perhaps significantly, by a disease that has gained
the upper hand and, in all likelihood, cannot be con-
quered.

Often dying people direct their anger at physicians
and other members of the health care team, whom they
feel have failed in their duty to save them. Anger may be
turned inward as well; many cancer patients focus their
fury on past bad habits and behaviors that they feel may
have triggered the disease.

Unfortunately your partner may turn his or her rage
upon the people who perhaps least deserve it: you and
other members of the family. Indeed your partner's anger may seem irrational to you, since the most trivial
upsets and even the most well-meaning gestures can set
it off.

As difficult as it may be, try to remember that the
anger phase of the coping process is a natural and
healthy one; it allows your partner to vent the deep,
inner pain that comes with a terminal diagnosis and
eventually get on with living the rest of his or her life.

What You Can Do to Help

Above all, don't take your partner's anger personally,
but try to understand the reasons behind it. Listen to
your partner's complaints carefully, even if they seem
irrational to you. Perhaps he or she becomes angry
when you insist on running his or her bath every night.
To you such a gesture signifies comfort and care. To
your partner it may seem as if you are trying to control
his or her behavior, or that you think he or she is inca-

pable of handling such personal matters on his or her own.

Bargaining

We've all done it: "If I pass this exam, I'll never ignore my studies again." "If I can make it to my desk without my boss seeing me, I swear I'll never oversleep again." "If I can just keep living, I'll be a better, kinder person—I promise." When we make promises like this, we're bargaining with ourselves, with God, or with the fates to let bygones be bygones, to start with a clean slate. In the future, you are saying, things will be different.

Bargaining with death for a few more days or weeks or years may seem to you to be a futile effort. But this attitude shows progress along the road to acceptance: Your partner now accepts that the prognosis is terminal, but still hopes there is some way to "get away" with a little more time.

What You Can Do to Help

Try not to ridicule the deals your partner makes with death; you'd be surprised at how often they work. In Chapter 7 you met Isabel, a woman with metastatic breast cancer who was determined to see her granddaughter, Emily, graduate from college. Three years later Emily is a senior and, although her grandmother is quite ill, there is every chance she'll make it to the ceremony in June.

On the other hand when your partner begins to lose more and more of the deals—when the treatment protocol fails as expected even though your partner didn't snap at you all day or forget to call her mother or smoke a single cigarette—you must be there to support her and explain that she is not to blame for her illness or for the poor prognosis.

Depression

In almost every other circumstance depression is a negative state of mind and soul, one that undermines and demeans the human spirit. When it comes to death and dying, however, it is a vital coping stage for both you and your partner to pass through, for it allows you both to come to terms with the true sad nature of the impending event.

There may be many reasons your partner feels depressed at this time. One of them, of course, is that he or she is facing his final months and realizes that time is running out. Another reason your partner may sink into depression is not what lies in the future but what has occurred in the past. Goals not accomplished, mistakes that were made, harsh words or acts that can never be taken back.

Eventually most dying people come out of their depression naturally, sparked by a renewed commitment to enjoying what is left of life. Others need professional counseling, even medication, to rise up from the depths of their sadness and grief.

What You Can Do to Help

Talk and listen to your partner as he or she reviews life with all its joys and regrets. Take advantage of this time to clear the proverbial decks of past misgivings and mistakes. Help your partner put his or her life into proper perspective by pointing out his or her positive accomplishments and attributes.

Most important, if your partner remains in a depressed state for more than a few weeks, make sure his or her physician and/or counselor is aware of the situation. In most cases there is no need for the last months of someone's life to be spent in misery.

Acceptance

In the best of all possible worlds death would be seen as a natural part of life, and terminally ill patients could approach their own deaths with a sense of completeness and peace. Unfortunately in our culture death is to be absolutely denied, no matter the cost, and it is rare for someone not to fight against it despite the insurmountable odds and the physical pain involved.

There are signs, however, that this insistence on life at all costs is beginning to change. More and more people —and their physicians—are recognizing that dying can be a positive, dignified, natural stage of life. At some point in the coping process your partner may come to terms with his or her own death and accept it as a spiritual release from a body that, because of cancer, can no longer sustain life.

What You Can Do to Help

The most important thing you can do at this point in the process is to accept your partner's own acceptance. You, too, have been waging a battle against your partner's illness, and it won't be any easier for you to give up than it will be for your partner. It may be you who is urging "just one more treatment" or who remains stuck in the denial or anger stage long after your partner has come to terms with the prognosis.

Does accepting that death is likely mean giving up and passively waiting for the end? Hardly. In fact accepting the inevitable is a very positive step, because it frees you and your partner to make important decisions and plans that may make it possible to live out the rest of the time you have together in the most satisfying and loving way possible.

Although it may seem morbid, a very healthy and healing way to begin the acceptance process is to discuss with your partner some of the important details about his or her death. Many people have very clear ideas about how they wish their body to be disposed of, how their funeral and memorial services should be conducted, and how they would like distant friends and family to be informed about their death. As soon as you both feel comfortable discussing these matters, arrangements can be made with the help of your partner's physician and/or hospital social worker.

In addition to these important details, your partner must make another decision, one that requires serious thought on his or her part as well as consideration and discussion among the entire health care team. That decision involves how your partner would like to live out the remaining months or weeks of his or her life.

UNDERSTANDING THE HOSPICE APPROACH

Many cancer patients facing a terminal prognosis choose to keep fighting, to use every medical option available to the very end. That is a valid choice, one that you must support if your partner feels that this is the best route to travel.

On the other hand, more and more people with cancer are choosing what are known as hospice programs that allow the individual to replace aggressive medical treatment with an approach that stresses comfort and peace. No longer is cure the goal, but rather the dying person works with doctors, nurses, and counselors to make the rest of his or her life as meaningful and pain-free as possible.

There are two basic types of hospices: independent hospices and hospital-associated hospice wards, each having its own strengths and weaknesses, depending on the needs of the dying person and the family.

Independent Hospices

These facilities are not connected with any hospital or medical center, but instead are staffed by private doctors, nurses, and social workers. They provide inpatient care, home care, counseling for patients and family members, and other wide-ranging services such as occupational therapy and nutritional counseling. The main drawback of an independent hospice is availability. Not only does each hospice have a limited number of beds, but not every community has access to an independent hospice. Fortunately, more and more communities are offering at-home hospice care and other hospice programs.

Hospital-Associated Hospices

Many hospitals sponsor their own hospice wards, separate sections of the hospital set aside to provide beds and services for dying patients. The best hospital-associated hospice wards are designed with the special needs of these patients and their families in mind. Furnishings are warm and cozy, the hustle and bustle of regular ward activity is kept to a minimum, and visiting hours are extremely flexible. More and more community hospitals are providing these services. Ask your partner's physician for more information.

Both types of hospices share the same basic goal: a dedication to the care and comfort of the cancer fighter and the physical and emotional support of his or her family. If you and your partner choose the hospice-program approach, you can rest assured that you won't be alone—advice and help will be available to you on a twenty-four-hour-a-day basis.

In fact by joining a hospice program you and your partner will be joining another team, similar in makeup to the health care team that helped your partner through the treatment phase. In many cases the teams may overlap. The physician in charge of your partner's hospice care will no doubt work in close consultation with your partner's primary physician, if that arrangement seems useful and appropriate to all concerned. You'll be introduced to a staff of nurses, one or more of whom will spend several hours a day with your partner at home or in the facility. A social worker will help coordinate your partner's financial, emotional, and medical needs as well as help other members of the family cope with the hospice arrangement.

Choosing a Hospice Approach

With help and advice from the health care team, you and your partner should sit together and talk about how each of you sees the coming weeks and months. Before you decide for or against a hospice approach, consider the following factors:

• *Your partner's prognosis and current condition.* Most hospices only accept patients who have been told they have six months or less to live. Your partner's physician will probably have to sign a document to that effect before your partner can be admitted into the program. However, there are exceptions. More and more hospices offer preliminary palliative-care programs for cancer patients whose prognosis is poor but still uncertain.

• *Your partner's wishes.* Clearly the hospice approach to death and dying is not for everyone. Your partner may want to continue to fight with every means available. Or he or she may feel more comfortable and secure—especially if pain is an issue—in a hospital setting. Some people feel strongly that dying at home would be too much of a burden on the family no matter how often or strongly they are told differently. Encourage your partner to talk to his or her doctor and counselor for objective advice, then respect your partner's wishes to the best of your ability.

• *Your own wishes.* It is important for you to realize before agreeing to an at home hospice approach that your responsibilities are likely to be much more extensive and the emotional involvement far greater than those you faced as a caregiver in the past. Carefully consider—with help and advice from your partner and a hospice counselor—whether or not you have the time, the energy, and the will to help your partner in this way.

If you decide you are unable to accept this commitment, do not feel guilty or ashamed. The hospice approach is not for every patient, nor is it for every caregiver. If your partner is committed to joining a hospice program, work together and with a social worker to involve another family member or close friend in your partner's care.

• *Your family's wishes.* Unless your partner chooses an inpatient hospice program, it is likely that he or she will live out most of his or her remaining months at home. Needless to say, the life of other family members living at home will undergo considerable emotional and practical changes that must be considered. Before you enter into this situation, you and your family should all sit down together and discuss the changes that may occur.

Among the many practical questions that should be addressed are the following:

1. Will the loved one with cancer have his or her own room? If your partner is also your spouse, it is likely that at some point you will no longer want to share a bed if either of you expects to get a full night's sleep.

2. Can the cancer patient stay alone when family

members go to work or school? Even during the critical treatment phases, it is likely that your partner was able to be left alone for several hours at a time. As his or her condition worsens, however, around-the-clock care may be necessary.

3. Will extra help be needed at home? If so, how will you pay for it? Can the family handle the extra expenses involved? Although many insurance policies, as well as Medicaid, will pay most of the hospice expenses, you must take your finances into consideration. Talk the matter over with a hospital or hospice social worker.

Although your first instinct may be to say, "Things will take care of themselves," it is far better to discuss these issues *before* they come up. That way each member of the family including the person with cancer will understand—and have time to accept—what is expected of him or her. This will help to avoid resentment and confusion in the future.

Even when major issues have been settled and family roles have been assigned, it is imperative that the lines of communication remain open. Both the cancer patient and other family members must feel able to voice their opinions and emotions freely during this very difficult period.

It is especially important for your partner to know that he or she can disagree or make reasonable demands without fearing that the family will reject him or her. Indeed as difficult as it may be at times, each family member should try to accommodate the changing needs of the cancer patient with love and acceptance. As discussed in Chapter 7, love and acceptance are as important to your partner as medical therapy.

Accepting the possibility that treatment will fail is an important aspect of coping with a cancer diagnosis, for both you and your partner. At the same time a positive diagnosis and successful treatment takes adjustment too. Cancer survivors and their caregivers may well look at life in the future very differently than those who have not yet been faced with such a fundamental challenge. Please read the "Afterword" to see what you and your partner can do to make the future as bright and full as possible.

Afterword:
Living Well as Survivors

The good news, as you and your partner may well discover, is that the fight against cancer can be won. As stated several times in this text, more and more people every day are declared cancer-free after treatment for one type of malignancy or another. Three million Americans now proudly proclaim their status as cancer survivors, and their ranks continue to grow.

These same triumphant survivors will admit, however, that the fight against cancer is never truly over—for either the cancer fighters or the caregivers. Although the first battle was won when the cancer was eradicated, many cancer survivors are surprised to find that many other skirmishes—emotional and physical—lie ahead.

Perhaps the most common problem faced by cancer survivors and their caregivers is the sense of isolation and "difference" from other people. Indeed the experience of fighting cancer has changed both you and your partner, and you are likely to see life from a different perspective from some of your friends and family who have not yet had to face a life-threatening illness in such a personal, intimate way. You may feel stronger and more ready to face problems, large and small, than other people in your life. Or you may consider yourself more vulnerable and less willing to take risks because you've seen how fragile life can be.

It is important that you recognize and accept these differences between you and your family circle before they interfere in a fundamental way with your relationships. Both you and your partner should attempt to share your new perspective in as open and honest a way as possible. Talk about what you've learned about life, death, and the fight against disease—your insights are an invaluable asset to any relationship you may form—without letting these subjects overwhelm your other interests and aspects of your personality.

Another long-term emotional side effect of a fight against cancer—even a thoroughly successful fight is fear—fear of what has occurred in the past and fear of a recurrence in the future. Indeed it is common for cancer survivors and/or their caregivers to suffer from nightmares about their past experiences with the disease or "daymares" about the cancer coming back. These fears are perfectly normal, especially during the first several years following the end of treatment. The longer your partner lives without a recurrence, the more these fears will fade into the background of your lives.

One way to hasten this process along is to realize that cancer will remain a part of your lives forever: Any long-term cancer survivor and any oncologist will tell you that it is impossible—and ultimately unhealthy—to put cancer behind you forever. Instead you and your partner should make every attempt to face that realization with optimism and commitment and use the very same emotional and physical resources that allowed you to fight the cancer to make your partner's future— and your own—as healthy and secure as possible.

Here are a few tips:

1. *Remain in a supportive environment.* The friends you and your partner made through your support groups during the treatment phase will remain invaluable sources of comfort and support in the years to come.

2. *Be vigilant about follow-up care for your partner.* No doubt your partner's physician has already told you both how important regular checkups are to the future of your partner's health. It is an unfortunate fact of life that recurrences of the same cancer may occur in your partner; in addition he or she may run a slightly higher risk of developing a new cancer than someone with no prior history of the disease. The primary physician treating your partner will provide a schedule of follow-up appointments (usually every three months for the first year, every six months for the second year, and once a year after that). Strongly encourage your partner to keep these appointments.

3. *Watch for signs and symptoms of cancer*—both in your partner and in yourself. As stated above, surviving cancer once will not immunize your partner against a recurrence or the development of a new cancer. Neither will helping someone fight cancer render *you* immune. It is important that you both remain alert to the signs and symptoms of cancer, perform regular self-exams of the breast if you are a woman and of the prostate if you

are a man, and visit your physician on a regular basis
for checkups.

According to the American Cancer Society, if you
have any of the following seven warning symptoms,
consult your physician as soon as possible:

> Changes in bowel or bladder habits
> A sore that does not heal
> Unusual bleeding or discharge
> Thickening or lump in a breast or elsewhere in
> your body
> Indigestion or swallowing difficulty
> Obvious change in a wart or mole
> Nagging cough or hoarseness

4. *Lead a healthy life.* No doubt you and your partner have developed a new appreciation for what many
of us take for granted: our health. Waking up feeling
refreshed, having enough energy to pursue our hobbies
and careers, opening our hearts and minds to the joy
and satisfaction that comes with friendship and family
love—none of this comes easily to a body that doesn't
receive proper nutrition or a mind/spirit overwhelmed
by stress.

There are several steps you and your partner can take
to ensure that the years to come are healthy ones:

• *Quit smoking.* Cigarette smoking is the number-
one risk factor, not only for the development of cancer
but for the other major killer in the Western world,
heart disease. If you do nothing else for your health this

year, stop smoking and encourage your partner to do so with you.

• *Eat a balanced diet.* Eating a high-fiber, low-fat diet will reduce your risk of developing cancer, heart disease, and a host of other conditions related to poor diet, including diabetes and hypertension. As well as reducing fat, it is important that you increase your intake of fruits and vegetables, which contain disease-fighting vitamins and minerals.

• *Exercise regularly.* Although lack of exercise has not yet been linked to increased cancer risk, the American Cancer Society recently added a sedentary lifestyle to its risk factors for heart disease, the nation's number-one killer. If you do not exercise at least three times a week for thirty minutes or more, you and your partner should create an exercise plan—with the help of your physicians—and stick to it.

• *Understand the mind-body connection.* As you learned in Chapter 7, sustained, unrelieved stress may play havoc with your body's ability to fight disease. It is essential that you understand and release the emotions and tension you hold within you. Some people find that meditation is the answer, others work out their emotions with exercise or through psychological counseling. Work with your partner and, if you choose, with your physician to find the best way for you to discover and make use of your own mind-body connection.

• *Enjoy yourselves.* You and your partner have fought and won a major battle against a formidable enemy. If you're like most cancer survivors, this experience has given you a new perspective on life, allowing you to see more clearly its fragility, its joys, and the hope that is implicit in the future. Revel in that future and all of its marvelous, as yet unknown possibilities.

Appendix 1: Resources

The *National Cancer Institute* (National Institutes of Health, Bethesda, MD 20205) is the federal government's agency for cancer research and control. Part of the National Institutes of Health (NIH) in Bethesda, Maryland, NCI conducts research on cancer prevention, diagnosis, treatment, and rehabilitation in its own laboratories. In addition to publishing informational material available to the public, the NCI has two important resources available to you and your partner:

• The *Cancer Information Service* (1-800-4-CANCER) can answer a wide variety of questions about causes of cancer, cancer prevention, specific types of cancer, and ways to detect, treat, and otherwise cope with the disease. Free booklets are available on these topics.

Besides giving out general information, CIS staff can refer people with cancer to local and regional hospitals and physicians that can provide first or second opinions or medical care. CIS can also refer patients to local organizations that provide support services, such as physical, occupational, and speech therapy; psychological counseling; support groups; home care; child care; meal preparation; transportation; and advice on financial aid.

• The *Physician Data Query (PDQ)* is NCI's computerized service for providing both doctors and patients with up-to-date information on cancer treatment. This database lists current treatment options for specific types of cancer at particular stages. It also notes what clinical trials are being conducted to test investigational therapies and where they are taking place. PDQ information can be obtained by calling the Cancer Information Service.

• *The NCI's Comprehensive Cancer Centers* are medical research facilities designed to investigate new methods of diagnosis and treatment of cancer patients. These centers have teams of experts working together on the most pressing and promising avenues of cancer research. They treat cancer patients, provide second opions, and try new treatments through clinical trials. In addition to the twenty comprehensive cancer centers, the NCI also supports research in about twenty-five hospitals across the country. Talk to your partner's physician and/or contact the NCI in Bethesda for a referral to one of the comprehensive or clinical cancer centers.

The *American Cancer Society* (National Headquarters, 1599 Clifton Road, N.E. Atlanta, GA 30329) is a national, voluntary organization that fights cancer through research, education, and patient service and rehabilitation programs. Nationwide the American Cancer Society (ACS) has about fifty-eight chartered divisions with about three thousand local units.

In addition to administering programs of research, medical grants, and clinical fellowships, the ACS provides information and counseling services for the cancer fighter and family. Its services include donating and/or loaning equipment such as sickroom supplies and hospital beds to cancer fighters at home, providing transportation to and from the hospital and in some cases lending social-work assistance and home health care. Some of ACS's outreach programs include the following:

- *I Can Cope* is a course designed to address the educational and psychological needs of people with cancer.
- *Reach to Recovery* offers emotional and physical support to women with breast cancer and their families.

In addition to these two major national organizations there are literally hundreds of smaller associations and institutions available to help cancer fighters and their families:

The *Encore* program, which provides counseling and rehabilitation to postoperative breast cancer patients, is conducted through local branches of the Young Women's Christian Association (YWCA). Check the white pages of your local phone book or the national office (Encore, National Board, 126 Broadway, New York, NY 10003).

The *Look Good, Feel Better* program is designed to help cancer patients deal with changes in their appearance resulting from chemotherapy or radiation treatment and is run in conjunction with the Cosmetic, Toiletry, and Fragrance Association Foundation and the National Cosmetology Association.

Let's Face It (Box 711, Concord, MA 01742) is a network of resources to help patients deal with facial disfigurements caused by surgery to treat head and neck cancers.

The *United Ostomy Association* (National Headquarters, 36 Executive Park, Suite 120, Irvine, CA 92714) is organized and administered by ostomates— people living with ostomies—to help other ostomy patients cope with the psychological and physical effects of their surgeries.

The *National Hospice Organization* (1901 Fort Myer Drive, Suite 901, Arlington, VA 22209, 703-243-5900) provides information about hospice care in general as well as the locations of services in different areas throughout the country.

The *Visiting Nurses Associations of America* (National Office, 3801 East Florida Avenue, Suite 206, Denver, CO 80210) will help you locate part-time nursing help for your partner at home.

The *Corporate Angel Network* (Building One, Westchester County Airport, White Plains, NY 10604) offers free air transportation to approved medical facilities for cancer patients and their families, subject to availability.

Your local library and bookstore are both vast resources for information about cancer and related subjects. Just a few of the literally hundreds of books that you and your partner may find helpful include:

Bricklin, Mark. *The Practical Encyclopedia of Natural Healing*. New York: Penguin Books, 1990.

Chase, Deborah. *Dying at Home with Hospice*. St. Louis: C. V. Mosby Company, 1986.

Dollinger, Malin, M.D., Ernest Rosenbaum, M.D., and Greg Cable. *Everyone's Guide to Cancer Therapy*. Toronto: Somerville House Books, Ltd., 1986.

Hollub, Arthur I., M.D. *The American Cancer Society Cancer Book: Prevention, Detection, Diagnosis, Treatment, Rehabilitation, Cure*. New York: Doubleday, 1986.

Hughes, Jennifer. *Cancer and Emotion*. New York: John Wiley & Sons, 1978.

Lindsay, Anne. *The American Cancer Society Cookbook*. New York: Hearst Books, 1988.

Little, Deobrah Whiting. *Home Care for the Dying*. New York: Doubleday, 1985.

Morra, Marion, and Eve Potts. *Choices: Realistic Alternatives in Cancer Treatment*. New York: Avon Books, 1987.

Morra, Marion, and Eve Potts. *Triumph: Getting Back*

to Normal When You Have Cancer. New York:
Avon Books, 1990.

Moyers, Bill. *Healing and the Mind.* New York: Doubleday, 1993.

Mullan, Fitzhugh, M.D., and Barbara Hoffman, J.D.
*Consumer Reports: Charting the Journey, An Al-
manac of Practical Resources for Cancer Survivors.*
New York: Consumers Union of the United States,
1990.

Simonton, O. Carl, Stephanie Matthews-Simonton and
James Creighton. *Getting Well Again: A Step-by-
Step, Self-Help Guide to Overcoming Cancer.* Bos-
ton: Houghton-Mifflin, 1978.

Winograd, Sarah. *Get Help, Get Positive, Get Well:
The Aggressive Approach to Cancer Therapy.*
Highland City, Fl.: Rainbow Books, 1992.

Appendix 2: Glossary

Acupressure: The use of finger pressure over various points on the body to treat symptoms or disease.

Adenocarcinoma: Cancer that arises from glandular tissues, such as cancers of the breast, lung, thyroid, colon, and pancreas.

Adenoma: A benign (nonmalignant) tumor that arises from glandular tissues.

Adjuvant chemotherapy: Chemotherapy used along with surgery or radiation therapy. It is usually given after all visible and known cancer has been removed by surgery or radiotherapy, but is sometimes given before surgery. Adjuvant chemotherapy is usually used in cases where there is a high risk of hidden cancer cells remaining and may increase the likelihood of cure.

Alopecia: Partial or complete loss of hair, often as a result of radiotherapy to the head or from certain chemotherapeutic agents.

Ambulatory infusion: The administration of chemotherapy by a small pump device that delivers anticancer drugs slowly and gradually. It is usually worn under clothes and allows patients to be treated at home and to participate in normal activities.

Analgesic: Any drug that relieves pain, ranging from mild pain relievers such as aspirin or ibuprophen to stronger drugs such as codeine and morphine.

Anemia: A condition in which there is less than the normal amount of hemoglobin or red blood cells in the blood. This may be due to bleeding, to lack of blood production by the bone marrow, or to the brief survival of blood already manufactured. Symptoms include fatigue, shortness of breath, and weakness.

Antibody: A protein made by the body's immune system in response to a specific foreign protein called an antigen. The antigen may result from an infection, a cancer, or some other source.

Antiemetics: Drugs given to prevent or minimize nausea and vomiting.

Aspiration: Removal of fluid or tissue, usually with a needle or tube, from a specific area of the body. This procedure may be done to obtain a diagnosis or to relieve symptoms.

Atrophy: A withering of a tissue or part of the body, which may result from a lack of use during prolonged bed rest or from pressure from an adjacent tumor.

Axilla: The armpit. Lymph glands in the armpit are called the axillary nodes.

Basal cell carcinoma: A form of skin cancer that grows very slowly and is curable in almost all cases by surgery or other local treatment.

Benign: A tumor that has no tendency to grow into

surrounding tissue or spread to other parts of the body. Under the microscope a benign tumor does not resemble cancer.

Biopsy: The surgical removal of a small portion of tissue for microscopic examination and diagnosis.

Bone marrow: A soft substance found within bone cavities. Marrow is composed of developing red cells, white cells, platelets, and fat. Some forms of cancer can be diagnosed by examining bone marrow.

Bone marrow examination: The process of removing bone marrow by withdrawing it through a needle for examination. It is usually withdrawn from the breastbone or the hipbone. The procedure is performed under local anesthesia and takes about ten minutes.

Bone scan: A picture of all the bones in the body taken about two hours after injection of a radioactive tracer. This test can help determine if cancer has spread to the bones.

Cancer: Uncontrolled cell proliferation that, when untreated, is fatal.

Carcinogen: A cancer-causing agent.

Carcinoma: A form of cancer that develops in the tissues covering or lining organs of the body such as the skin, uterus, lung, or breast. Eighty to 90 percent of all cancers are carcinomas.

Cell cycle: Each cell in the body, including a cancer cell, goes through several stages every time it divides. Various anticancer drugs affect the cell at different stages of this cycle.

Cells: The fundamental unit, or building blocks, of human tissue.

Centigray: A unit of measurement of radiation therapy.

Cervix: The lower portion of the uterus, which protrudes into the vagina. The Pap test is designed to check this area for cancer.

Chemotherapy: The treatment of cancer by chemicals (drugs) designed to kill cancer cells or stop them from growing.

Chromosomes: The fundamental strands of genetic material (DNA) that carry all our genes.

Colonscopy: A procedure to inspect and biopsy the rectum and colon by means of a long, flexible fiberoptic telescope.

Colony-stimulating factor (CFS): A substance that stimulates the growth of bone marrow cells. Current clinical trials are using CFS to try to increase the dosage of chemotherapy that can be given safely.

Colostomy: An artificial opening, either temporary or permanent, in the abdominal wall created so that feces drains from the colon into a bag. Colostomies are often necessary after the removal of a diseased section of the large intestine.

Colposcopy: Inspection of the cervix with special binocular magnifying instruments to detect cancer with the use of a stain.

Combination chemotherapy: The use of several anticancer drugs at the same time.

Computerized tomography (CT scan): X ray that creates cross-section images of the body that may show cancer or metastases earlier than other imaging methods.

Cyst: A fluid-filled, usually benign, sac of tissue.

Cystitis: An inflammation of the bladder, often caused

by chemotherapy or radiation treatments as well as by infection with bacteria. Symptoms include a burning sensation while urinating or frequent urge to urinate.

Cytology: The microscopic examination of cells.

Debulking: The reduction in size of a tumor by either surgery or chemotherapy.

Differentiation: The process of maturation of a cell line of cancer cells.

Diuretics: Drugs that increase the elimination of water and salts in the urine.

Dysphagia: Difficulty in swallowing, a sensation of food sticking in the throat.

Edema: Swelling caused by the accumulation of fluid within tissues.

Electron beam: A form of radiotherapy in which the beam does not penetrate completely through the body as ordinary X rays do. It is primarily used to treat skin cancer or lesions beneath the skin.

Endocrine glands: Glands that secrete hormones to control bodily functions.

Endometrial carcinoma: A cancer of the inner lining of the uterus, called the endometrium.

Enteral feeding: Administration of liquid food through a tube inserted into the stomach or intestine.

Epidural: The space just outside the spinal cord. Plastic catheters may be inserted in the space to deliver anesthetics or morphine for pain control.

Esophagitis: Soreness and inflammation of the esophagus due to infection, toxicity from radiation therapy or chemotherapy, or from physical injury.

Estrogen: The female sex hormone produced primarily by the ovaries.

Estrogen-receptor (ER) assay: A test that determines whether the breast cancer in a particular patient is stimulated by the hormone estrogen.

Excision: Surgical removal of tissue.

Fine-needle aspiration: A method to obtain small bits of tissue for diagnosis, in which a small needle is inserted through the skin directly into a tumor and a sample of tissue is drawn up into the needle.

Grade of tumor: A way of describing tumors by their appearance under the microscope. Low-grade tumors are slow to grow and spread, while high-grade tumors grow and spread rapidly.

Hematologist: A physician who specializes in blood diseases.

Hematuria: Blood in the urine.

Histology: The appearance of tissues under the microscope.

Hormonal anticancer therapy: A form of therapy that takes advantage of the tendency of some cancers to stabilize or shrink if certain hormones are either administered or withdrawn.

Hospice: A facility and philosophy of care that stress comfort, peace of mind, and the control of symptoms rather than cure, usually when no further anticancer therapy is available and life expectancy is considered short.

Hyperthermia: Increased body temperature often provoked by the use of special devices as a way of treating cancer, usually in conjunction with radiation therapy.

Hysterectomy: Surgical removal of the ovaries.

Immune system: The body mechanisms that resist and fight disease.

Immunotherapy: A method of cancer therapy that sitmulates the body's own defense mechanisms to attack cancer cells.

Incontinence: The inadvertant loss of urine or feces due to the loss of nerve or muscle control.

Inflammation: The triggering of the immune system causing defensive white blood cells to pour into the affected tissues, causing redness, heat, pain, and swelling.

Informed consent: A legal standard that defines how much a patient must know about the potential benefits and risks of therapy before agreeing to it.

Infusion: Administration of fluids or medications into a vein or artery over a period of time.

In situ: A very early stage of cancer in which the tumor is localized to one area.

Interferon: A natural substance produced in response to infections. Interferon has been created artificially and used to treat cancer.

Intravenous: The administration of drugs or fluids directly into a vein.

Invasive cancer: Cancer that spreads to the healthy tissue surrounding the original cancer site.

Large-cell carcinoma: A type of cancer of the lung.

Localized: A cancer confined to the site of origin without evidence of spread.

Lumbar puncture (spinal tap): Removal of spinal fluid for examination that involves numbing the skin of the back with a local anesthetic and placing a needle into the numbed area to remove the spinal fluid.

Lumpectomy: The removal of a breast cancer and the surrounding tissue without removing the entire breast. It is usually followed by radiation and/or chemotherapy.

Lymph nodes: Oval-shaped organs roughly the size of peas, located throughout the body, that act as the immune system's first line of defense against infections and cancer. Lymph nodes produce infection-fighting white blood cells as well as filter out bacteria, foreign substances, and cancer cells.

Lymphatic system: The system of lymph nodes and the lymphatic vessels that connect them.

Lymphocytes: White blood cells responsible for the production of antibodies and for the direct destruction of invading organisms or cancer cells.

Malignant: An adjective meaning "cancerous"; malignant cells tend to sink roots into surrounding tissues as well as break off and spread elsewhere.

Metastasis: The spread of cancer from one part of the body to another by way of the lymph system or bloodstream. Cells in the new cancer are like those in the original tumor.

Monoclonal antibodies: Highly specific antibodies, usually manufactured in a laboratory, that react to a specific cancer antigen or are directed against a specific type of cancer.

Magnetic resonance imaging (MRI): A method of creating three-dimensional images of the body using a magnetic field and radio waves rather than X rays.

Mucositis: Inflammation of the mucous membranes resulting in cold-sore-like lesions in the mouth, caused by chemotherapy.

Necrosis: The distintegration of tissue caused by some physical or chemical agent or by the lack of a blood supply.

Neoplasm: A new abnormal growth, of either benign or malignant nature.

Nerve block: Pain relief effected by the numbing of a nerve with a local anesthetic.

Neuropathy: Malfunction of a nerve, causing numbness or weakness, often resulting from anticancer treatment.

Neurotoxicity: Toxic effects of chemotherapy on the nervous system.

Oncogenes: Specific stretches of cellular DNA that, when triggered, contribute to the transformation of normal cells into malignant ones.

Oncologist: A physician who specializes in cancer therapy. There are surgical, radiation, pediatric, gynecological, and medical oncologists. The term *oncologist* alone generally refers to medical oncologists, who are internists with expertise in chemotherapy and the handling of the general medical problems that arise during the disease.

Opportunistic infections: Common microorganisms that do not ordinarily cause infections in healthy people but that can cause serious disease in those whose immune systems are compromised by the cancer itself or the therapy used to treat it.

Ostomy: A surgically created opening in the skin leading to an internal organ, for purposes of drainage.

Palliative: Treatment that aims to improve well-being,

relieve symptoms, or control the growth of cancer, but not primarily intended or expected to produce a cure.

Parenteral nutrition: Artificial feeding by the intravenous administration of nutrients.

Pathology: Study of disease through the examination of body tissues, organs, and materials.

Polyp: A growth that protrudes from mucous membranes, which may be found in the nose, ears, mouth, lungs, vocal cords, uterus, cervix, rectum, bladder, and intestine.

Potassium: A mineral in the body that is often lost during illness, especially with diarrhea.

Primary tumor: The place where a cancer first starts to grow.

Prognosis: A statement about the likely outcome of disease in a particular patient based on all available information about the type of tumor, its stage, treatment options, expected results, and other factors.

Prosthesis: An artificial replacement of a body part, such as a leg or breast.

Protocol: A cancer treatment program, including dosages and formulas for any drugs to be administered.

Radiation oncologist: A physician who specializes in the use of radiation to treat cancer.

Radiation therapy: The use of radiation from X-ray machines, cobalt, radium, or other sources for control or cure of cancer.

Radical mastectomy: Removal of the entire breast along

with underlying muscle and the lymph nodes of the armpit.

Radioactive implant: A source of high-dose radiation that is placed directly into and around a cancer to kill the cancer cells.

Radiologist: A physician specializing in the use of X rays as well as other imaging techniques (e.g., computerized tomography or magnetic resonance imaging) to diagnose disease.

Recurrence: The reappearance of a disease after treatment had apparently effected a cure.

Regression: The shrinkage of a cancer, usually as the result of therapy.

Remission: The partial or complete shrinkage of cancer occurring as a result of therapy.

Risk factors: The habits or conditions that promote the development of cancer.

Sarcoma: A cancer of supporting or connective tissue such as cartilage, bone, muscle, or fat. Sarcomas are often highly malignant. They account for about 2 percent of all human cancers.

Second-look surgery: Surgery to determine if aggressive chemotherapy and/or radiation therapy has been successful.

Sigmoidoscopy: An examination of the rectum and lower colon with a hollow lighted tube called a sigmoidoscope. It is used to detect colon polyps and cancer and to find the cause of bleeding.

Sphincter: A circular muscle that tightens around an organ or cavity to close it and to regulate the flow of material.

Sputum: Material coughed up from the lungs.

Squamous cell carcinoma: Cancer arising from the skin or the surfaces of other structures, such as the mouth, cervix, or lungs.

Staging: A process of determining how large or serious a cancer has become and/or how far it has spread. Staging involves physical examination, blood tests, X rays and other imaging techniques, and often surgery.

Stoma: A surgically created opening in the skin for elimination of body wastes.

Suppository: A way to administer medications by absorbing the drug into a wax preparation, then inserting it into the rectum or vagina.

Ulcer: A sore resulting from corrosion of normal tissue by some irritating substance, such as chemicals, infection, or cancer.

Ultrasound: The use of high-frequency sound waves to create an image of the inside of the body.

Undifferentiated: A tumor that does not resemble tissues of the organ in which the cancer orginates. These tumors tend to grow and spread faster than well-differentiated tumors.

Well-differentiated: A tumor that resembles normal tissue from the same organ.

White blood cells: Cells in the blood that fight infection.

Index